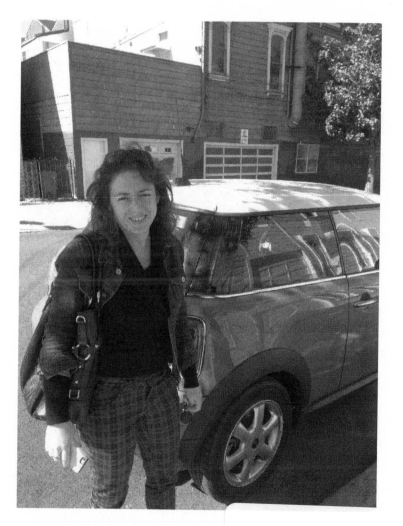

Introduction

Rachel Eleah Roisman, M.D., M.P.H., a board-certified internist and public health doctor, was 42 years old when she died. At age 39, she had been diagnosed with a rare, aggressive cancer – mesenchymal chondrosarcoma. This is the blog she wrote during those years. It's funny, sad, and oddly inspiriting. We have left it exactly as she wrote it, without any editorial changes or corrections. Its spirit is suggested by these excerpts, from the beginning and end of those years. The references to J are to her husband, whom she loved passionately.

From her first post, recording her diagnosis and noting that it is "something like less than 1% of chondrosarcomas, which are hardly common":

> *Here's a conversation J and I have had at least three times in the past 24 hours.*

J: "So, you have lung cancer"

Me: "Actually, it's more accurate to think of it as bone cancer, in the lung."

J: "Seriously, what the fuck, can't you just do something normal?"

It's a fair point, since when did I go from being a horse to a zebra?

And from May 2016, three months before she died:

Sooooo overdue for a post – apologies! The whole "chemo not working, more brain mets, seizures, whole-brain xrt, home hospice, etc." has really cramped my style! . . . .

The good news is that I happen to be the only person who has ever looked better thanks to the miracles of high-dose steroids. This is all really helping with my hospice as money-maker plan. There has got to be a big market for some hospice-based pornography and I plan to exploit it!

As these excerpts indicate, Rachel had a profound and unique sense of humor and an unblinking view of life and the world. She was irreligious and rejected every form of cant. She enjoyed good food, travel, art, movies, swimming, and theater. She deeply loved her husband, family members, her cadre of amazing friends, the San

3

Francisco Giants, and the two dogs she and her husband had adopted. She did not want to be sick and she certainly did not want to die young, but she also did not want to be kept alive by extraordinary measures. When it became clear that the surgery, chemotherapy, and radiation had done what they could, she went into hospice care. She found better news there – outings, usually related to food; release from the obligation to floss her teeth (as she wrote, in home hospice care, "acceptable evening dental care = a root beer float followed by minty ice cream"). She regretted that she'd fallen behind in her reading of "The Economist" (really: Us Weekly). She died in her home, in the loving companionship of her husband, her best friend, her parents, and her two dogs.

Rachel's all-too-short life was extraordinary. She grew up in Washington, D.C., where she attended the Barbara Chambers Children's Center and Georgetown Day School. She then earned her B.S. at Dartmouth College and her M.D. from Johns Hopkins School of Medicine.

At Dartmouth, she completed a fellowship studying birth control practices and providing reproductive health counseling in India. Between college and medical school, she worked as a community organizer addressing food insecurity in Oakland, CA. While at Hopkins, she led Medical Students for Choice and spent a year at the Health Research Group of Public Citizen in Washington, D.C. She served rotations with the Public Health

Department of Baltimore, MD and the Native Alaskan Health Service.

Rachel did her residency in internal medicine at the Primary Care Program of the San Francisco General Hospital. She then held a fellowship in Occupational and Environmental Medicine and earned her Master's degree in Public Health at the University of Washington. Always committed to health equity and public service, she was part of the emergency medical efforts that responded to Hurricane Katrina in New Orleans and the 2010 earthquake in Haiti; she also provided medical assistance in Uganda and Nicaragua.

After her fellowship at the University of Washington, she joined the California Environmental Protection Agency and then the California Department of Public Health, where she led investigations of work-related injury and illness, focusing on some of the most vulnerable workers in California. In addition, she helped to establish a unique training program focused on underserved workers for residents in occupational medicine at UCSF, where she was a beloved mentor to many trainees. She worked clinically at the Veterans Administration hospital in San Francisco. She volunteered at Berkeley Animal Care Services, from which she and J adopted Cleo and Frankie.

Rachel left behind a treasure trove of memories of an extraordinary human being. Her dedication to helping others and to helping to create a more just world left indelible imprints on the lives of those of us who knew and loved her. Of her many attributes, her gift for friendship and love, her humor, and her life-affirming attitude may be most striking. Her blog – Cancerwithoutwalkathons – so conveys her spirit that we want to share it with the world in the hope that it will provide to others both comfort and inspiration.

Florence Wagman Roisman
Anthony Zell Roisman

October 1st, 2017

January 23, 2013

I want you to have visible symptoms

"Or I can't take care of you because you're healthier than I am."

Yeah, it's weird not having symptoms and being told you've got an absurdly rare and highly problematic potentially metastatic cancer. Fortunately, we're still at the point where I think it's funny when J says shit like that to me.

For those of you not privy to the backstory:

In June I was diagnosed with unilateral iritis, presumably idiopathic and completely random. I had 2 other episodes in the fall that resolved before I even saw the opthamologist again. In December, when it happened again, I went back to optho because I figured I needed a diagnosis since recurrent iritis warrants a work-up. The blood work (RPR, HLAB27, ACE) was normal but since the ACE was just past the normal range and I've got an aunt with sarcoid and a brother with Crohn's I figured there's a little autoimmunity floating around in my genes so I requested a CXR. The CXR showed a 5cm mostly calcified mass thought to be a tuberculoma. Now didn't I feel foolish for having my friends read my PPDs all those years? So then I was off to TB clinic to be a special patient of Dr. C! The CT scan was more suggestive of a benign hamartoma than something infectious. As much as I enjoyed my post lung biopsy conscious sedation nap, I knew it was a bad sign when "we'll have results in 2 days" turned into "we don't know what it is so we're sending the slides out." I wonder how many people can say that it was the pathologist who was the one to give them their cancer diagnosis? Isn't that why people go into pathology, to avoid having to say that sort of thing to people? But I was in the neighborhood so decided to ambush the pathologist and he kindly agreed to show me the slides. "These cells are cartilage, and these cells are malignant." I like to think I was the first person to whom he had to give an in-person cancer diagnosis.

But seriously, mesenchymal chondrosarcoma? Something like less than 1% of chondrosarcomas, which are hardly common. And don't google it...just don't. Here's a conversation J and I have had at least three times in the past 24 hours,

J: "So, you have lung cancer"

Me: "Actually, it's more accurate to think of it as bone cancer, in the lung."

J: "Seriously, what the fuck, can't you just do something normal?"

It's a fair point, since when did I go from being a horse to a zebra?

Next steps, PET scan tomorrow, meet with CT surgeon next week (he "guaranteed" me that there was nobody better to do the surgery than he - when I said that I was going to want to go to the local tertiary care center for evaluation in addition to my HMO which we will slyly refer to as "K"), and medical oncology next week.

January 24, 2013

One foot in

J's convinced I'm going to die, and leave him alone. He's already imagining that things we do together we are doing for the last time! It's making me feel a little not present. Which is all the more odd since I'm still asymptomatic.

We had a brief disagreement the other day when he said "I wish this were happening to me rather than you" and I said "I wish this were happening to me rather than you" and he said "I wish this were happening to me rather than you" and I said "well, it's not actually up to us, and it's happening to me." It turns out that's a great way to end a conversation. But the reality is, we both know it's easier to be the one who is sick than the one who is not so neither one of us is actually being selfless.

January 25, 2013

Let's just hope it's benign

Hmm, someone not quite getting the picture. We're kind of past the "benign" stage.

Off to a beer festival today. Not sure that bad news + unlimited etoh is a good combination. Update to follow.

Had the PET scan yesterday - did not actually realize what a PET scan was until I had it. It wasn't full body which doesn't make sense to me - I do have bones all over, right? The fun part is waiting 4 days for the results. I tried to trick the technicians into showing me the images cause I figured I could at least tell if there was something asymmetric, but they didn't fall for it!

J's new favorite thing whenever I inquire about doing anything is to say "what's the worst that will happen? It gives you cancer?"

I'm not convinced that his reaction to this is actually healthy.

January 26, 2013

I have really bad news

The BBQ placed we want to go to for lunch is closed on Sunday.

J and I have since discussed perhaps being a bit more selective about when, and in what context, we use that phrase.

January 29, 2013

Apparently I'm a really shitty doctor

If I believed in God, or karma, I might think that I'm being punished for practicing medicine by the "common things being common" mantra. The next time I see a patient, which may also be the last time I see a patient (morbid? I'll give you morbid, the oncologist doesn't even want to do chemo!), I think I'll try to get MRIs on everyone with hangnails, just in case the hangnail is a paraneoplastic manifestation of some sort of rare cancer! I'm going to try to admit the people with ankle sprains to medicine "for further workup."

I don't think I've provided much of a clinical update of late, so here goes:

PET scan showed the lesion in the lung plus a lesion in the left ilium (likely the primary) plus a spot in the right femoral head plus a 3cm lesion somewhere in the abdomen - all concerning for metastatic disease. The oncologist wants to biopsy one of those lesions just to make sure that everything is as shitty as it seems like it is. He is also suggesting that we see how fast things are growing by repeating the cxr in a month. His general suggestion is that if things aren't moving quickly, just chill, because chemo isn't likely to help much and surgery is going to be both unpleasant and not super useful. If things are moving quickly, than might as well do chemo, b/c things look so shitty anyway. Either way, the best case scenarios he paints were things like "I've got a patient with an angiosarcoma who was still alive 10 years later and

11

we didn't do chemo!" He is also suggesting that since new drugs are in development one never knows if a treatment or cure is just around the corner! That is seriously one of the most depressing things I have ever heard in my entire life. I could barely contain my desire to ask him if he was just blowing smoke up my ass, which I've never had anyone do before, but it seems like it would feel exactly how that conversation with him went.

Next steps - ice cream at least once a day, bone scan (mostly just for the heck of it in case it finds something the PET didn't) and potential biopsy of one of these other lesions, pending IR's input. Also, I've now got chest CTs and CXR from now and a month ago so the radiologist can see if the tumor has grown much. Oh yeah, and I also dropped out of work. I'm not officially on medical leave or disability but I guess I'll figure that out in the next few weeks. Suddenly I'm feeling like a genius for having a longterm disability policy!

The surgeons are more than happy to remove the lesions in my lung and ilium. Lung surgery sounds like a breeze (unless they get in there and find out that the tumor is attached to the SVC) - ortho surgery not so much fun - one option is a hemipelvectomy which leaves me with no hip joint, a leg that is 3" shorter, terrible function, and year of recovery! All I can think about are my boots, which apparently I will only need to wear on one leg, at least the ones with 3" heels. The other option is less drastic, scoop out the lesion, burn the surrounding bone, fill it in with cement, +/- hip replacement, and I am on crutches for 4-6 weeks, may have a limp, probably won't need a cane, and overall have decent function. I don't even know what surgery to remove the abdominal lesion would be like since it's not yet clear where it is - CT scan done today (the CT surgeon asked if I minded having another chest CT to go with the CT of the abdomen/pelvis since it was not really necessary and a big radiation dose - I pointed out that I should be so lucky as to worry about longterm consequences of radiation exposure!). But the oncologist is not suggesting surgery at this point.

If making snarky comments about my impending demise suddenly goes out of fashion this blog is gonna be kaput.

Oh, also, I'm trying to get my path sent to Dana Farber for review. And my request to be referred to the UCSF sarcoma guy was met by resistance! The oncologist said that they don't refer out if they have someone in-house, and they have a sarcoma expert in Santa Clara. I pointed out that I am not a 90 yo trying to have my gall bladder removed at UCSF and that as a young, healthy person with an absurdly rare cancer with a terrible prognosis, this is exactly the sort of thing that justifies the existence of places of UCSF. I really wanted to ask him what Kaiser does to him if he makes that referral because I cannot believe that any reasonable oncologist would think that it was not appropriate for someone in my situation to go see an uber-specialist. Nobody goes to work at Kaiser because they want to treat rare shit. I have an appt in a few weeks so I really don't give a shit if Kaiser approves it, but it is a point of pride to "win" this argument.

January 29, 2013

My first cancer boon!

My $20 was handed back to me after she asked if I had a history of cancer - apparently you don't have to pay for copies of your imaging if you have cancer!

January 30, 2013

So much less depressed!

J feels so much less depressed right now that he expects me to rub his feet tonight!

I realize that may not seem like good news to the average reader but it really is!

Up until this point, he has really been stuck in the first stage of grief - binge drinking.

Now if I can just get him to stop referring to me as "cancer lady." Or "cans," for short...

Not clear if our spring training training plans are still a reality. We're supposed to leave in a month. Pitchers and catchers report in less than 2 weeks! I did briefly google "what do I get from the SF Giants if I have cancer" - do I qualify for the Make-a-Wish Foundation???? If it's like those carnival rides and I just need to be no taller than Yosemite Sam to get in I'm golden!

January 30, 2013

Things J has said to me while hugging me

This one may need to be updated on a regular basis.
So far we have:

---

me: "you feel so good"

J: "you feel like cancer"

---

me: "I love you"

J: "I will probably never forget you"

---

me: "I'm going to get ice cream."

J: "Don't pork out on me; we don't yet know if you're doing chemo."

That one wasn't actually said while hugging.

January 30, 2013

My heart and my head

are totally in the right place when I tell J to wake me up in the middle of the night if he is sad - but apparently my subconscious is not on the right page because the past few times he has done this I've said "there, there, let's talk about this later when I'm not sleeping."

J says that he wants to rip my cancer out and poop on it.

That does remind me of a clinical trial...

January 31, 2013

Less awkward than one might think

It really was less awkward than one might think to have a former co-intern do a breast exam on me today. Since my body is clearly not doing me any favors these days it's pretty easy to just give it up to medical evaluation/intervention. I had my first mammogram (I really wanted to be wearing a tshirt that said "I believe in the USPSTF!" so that people wouldn't just think I was there as an asymptomatic, low-risk, woman wanting a screening mammogram at age 38). FYI, mammograms are really annoying. They take a while and involve squishing your breasts into all sorts of weird and awkward positions. Then I had an ultrasound - this whole thing is because of a mass/lymph node seen on CT that did not light up on PET scan and that everyone, including the breast surgeon, seems to think is not much of anything. But since there is a palpable mass on exam they went through all of this. The ultrasound was done initially by a tech but then the radiologist came in and low and behold my former co-intern! Evs. Good news is he didn't think it was anything either - a lymph node and not a scary one. This is actually the first time that a test hasn't resulted in worse news.

I saw the eye doctor this morning - remember that whole iritis thing that started this mess? I told the eye doctor that nobody other than me, and perhaps him, gives a shit about the iritis. Apparently this is just a total coincidence that I have a rare presentation of an absurdly rare cancer and I have an unusually recurrent idiopathic iritis. And it is hard not to wonder what would have happened had I not requested the cxr for the iritis work-up? When would this have been found? When the lung mass eroded into my SVC? I can't imagine that would have been a gentle presentation.

I also ran into the thoracic surgeon on the street which was very neighborly! He was not subtle about thinking it was odd that the oncologist is not inclined to do chemo or surgery. So he plans to talk to ortho onc. and discuss further.

Oh, and good news, I think, CXR today and the lung mass is no larger than it was 12/24 - that's good, right? But I don't know if that's actually good news or if it's just not really bad news.

Next steps: I've asked that the path go to Dana Farber (tho slides are still at UCSF so this might take a while), I have a

17

bone scan Monday, and I see Kaiser "sarcoma expert" next Thursday. This whole thing is a full time job! On the plus side, I do feel that I'm getting my money's worth from Kaiser - well, except for the not referring me out thing. I was thinking about seeing if I can get a monthly parking pass which can't possibly be more expensive than what we've been paying for parking.

It has now been more than 4 hours since I had a piece of chocolate - gotta go.

February 2, 2013

I have syphilis

And those were the last words I heard of the Lifetime movie "She's Too Young" before J came in and said "I forbid you to continue watching that." Apparently, I'm not supposed to have sunk quite to that level.

The worst part?

I'd already seen the movie.

February 3, 2013

Cry me a river

You know how every song on the radio sounds like it's about you when you've been through a breakup? I kind of had that experience yesterday, but the cancer version.

Patients I saw at the VA:

1. 60 something yo Vietnam Vet who just started chemo and can't sleep and his PTSD symptoms are acting up

2. 90 yo with metastatic prostate cancer (and bladder cancer as an added bonus)

3. 60 yo with NSCLC and now neutropenic fever after his most recent round of chemo.

4. 50 yo smoker with a cough x 4-6 weeks and now a new mass on his CXR! When I said "it may be something that requires a biopsy to make sure it's not cancer," he said "that must hurt a lot," and I said "actually, I had one 2 weeks ago and it's not that bad."

Ever since I was hospitalized with that MRSA abscess during residency I swore that I would not let my own medical experiences make me a more compassionate doctor. But damn it, I think I was nicer yesterday than I normally would have been!

Bone scan today, path off to Dana Farber, oncology appt on Thursday, and ilium biopsy scheduled for 2/14. I hear all the kids are trying to arrange bone biopsies for their moist, humorous, lovers (MI shout out!) this valentine's day.

February 4, 2013

Best cancer zinger...so far!

Dear Dr. xxx,

I was notified by yyy that you indicated a need to be out for your own serious health condition. While you are not eligible for FML, we will need documentation to support your need to be out. I am attaching the documents that have been mailed to the address that we have on file. Please do let me know if you have any questions at all.

zzz, HR Generalist

"Dear zzz, thank you for your kind words during these difficult times...."

I wanted to say "comforting" but J thought that was too much.

February 5, 2013

It's official

Path was reviewed by pathologist at Dana Farber - it is mesenchymal chondrosarcoma - confirming me as an unusual presentation of an absurdly rare malignancy! I really hope I get to be listed as a co-author on the case report.

"Many thanks for asking me to look at the needle biopsy of this physician's lesion in the upper lobe of the right lung. I note the radiologic evidence of coexistent lesions in the pancreas and left iliac bone. I agree entirely with your suggested diagnosis. Indeed the biopsy shows characteristic cytoarchitectural features of mesenchymal chondrosarcoma, in context most likely metastatic. The lesion consists of cytologically quite monomorphic small rounded cells with a high N/C ratio, arranged around prominent thin-walled, mainly slit-like vascular channels, adjacent to which there is a nodule of well differentiated cartilaginous tissue. Unfortunately, the behavior of these lesions cannot be predicted reliably on morphologic grounds and there is no applicable grading scheme in this regard. In particular, there is no correlation between the extent of the round cell component and clinical behavior. While some of these lesions may pursue a very indolent course, sometimes giving rise to metastases 15 or 20 years later, others are associated with a much more rapidly progressive clinical evolution."

February 6, 2013

Ok, now I'm starting to get annoyed

Spoke with 2 surgeons (thoracic, ortho onc.) - both of whom defer to the oncologist but assume that the plan will be to do chemo, then surgery, then more chemo. And I should see the general surgeon who does sarcoma stuff to discuss having the pancreatic lesion removed. And no biopsies are necessary since all these lesions are clearly related.

Spoke with the first oncologist who favored not doing anything since these tumors are normally slow growing (in comparison to breast/lung/etc. since they are fast growing in comparison to other chondrosarcomas), chemo doesn't do much, AND I may live long enough for a cure to come along. And biopsy the ilium lesion so that we know that all these lesions are related.

Spoke with the second oncologist who suggests surgery to take out all the lesions - left hip, right femur (tiny little spot), pancreatic tail, lung, a dash of XRT, then maybe chemo but probably not since chemo sucks and isn't going to do much. This guy was also promoting the "live long enough for a cure to come along" plan - which I've got to tell you is not actually that reassuring. He also said, no reason to biopsy the ilium lesion and it may seed the cancer elsewhere.

I asked the 2nd oncologist if my case had been discussed at tumor board - mostly because I wondered if any of these people were talking amongst themselves since they're all making completely different suggestions - and he dismissed tumor board since it's just a bunch of doctors sitting around saying what they think.

Uhm, isn't that what it's supposed to be? And if you don't respect the opinions of the doctors coming to tumor board perhaps you should stop inviting them and bring in some people who know what they're talking about? I didn't realize that the concept of people sitting around discussing cases and throwing out ideas was a bad one.

2nd oncologist also suggested I see hepatobiliary team regarding pancreatic lesion. I mentioned that ortho onc. had suggested I see sarcoma surgeon for this. Oncologist said "well, that's up to you, whether you want to see someone who deals with these sorts of cancers or someone who does a lot of pancreatic surgery." I said "I want to see the person who is going to do the best job of removing a sarcoma from my pancreas, if we decide that's the best thing to do! I don't want to go see 2 surgeons for this. Can't you all tell me who is most experienced dealing with this sort of thing?!?!?"

I can only imagine what a nightmare this would be for someone without a medical background. You'd end up choosing the treatment plan based on which physician you like the best.

I did like oncologist #2, don't get me wrong, though I was not encouraged that he seemed to know as much about treatment for this as I do, and he showed me abstracts from relevant studies and I when I asked follow-up questions he said "well, I've only seen the abstract, I haven't seen the full article."

Oncologist #2 was also reluctant to refer me to an academic center. His explanation was that he didn't see any reason for it since "nobody has seen a lot of these tumors" and they only refer if there's a treatment Kaiser can't offer.

I explained that at this point I'd be happy to see an oncologist who has treated ONE PERSON with this malignancy (neither Kaiser oncologist has EVER TREATED ANYONE WITH IT - and just to be clear, this 2nd oncologist is the Kaiser "sarcoma expert"). I finally asked him what happens to him if he requests the approval because I cannot understand how any reasonable physician would deny my request. He couldn't answer that question. In the end, he seemed convinced and said he would discuss it with my primary oncologist. But after the appointment he called me back and said that he spoke with my primary oncologist and they think I should just file a grievance with Kaiser to approve this referral. Which really sounded like "we don't think it's unreasonable but we can't make the referral for some really weird reason that we can't tell you about such as a)it makes us look bad to Kaiser b)they dock our pay c)we can no longer call ourselves experts d)it hurts our egos…" Regardless, I made the complaint to Kaiser and I'm waiting on the outside appt and will go regardless of what Kaiser says. Point of pride at convincing them to approve this be damned.

Next steps: go to academic center, get input from them on 1)whether biopsy of ilium lesion is warranted - so J will probably have to come up with another Vday present for me since we'll likely delay bx this until we get outside input.

2)different oncologist at Kaiser who is going to listen to outside suggestions cause now I don't trust current oncologists' judgment since they won't let me get a 2nd opinion

3)chemo, surgery, XRT???

Just a shout-out to all those people who are keeping my body fat up with your numerous, delicious, thoughtful presents of cookies, chocolates, etc. I feel compelled to tell you that I don't actually look like I have cancer, and with these gifts I may be moving in the direction of becoming the world's first morbidly obese metastatic cancer patient, but I do greatly appreciate everything everyone has been doing for us and both J and I feel very, very loved and taken care of by our friends and family.

Oh shit, the walk-a-thon is about to start and my cancer ribbon needs to be ironed, gotta go.

February 12, 2013

Gentle Readers

Dear Gentle Readers, the outpouring of love and support from you all has been fantastic and we greatly appreciate all the gifts that are being sent this way. Particularly now that chemo seems quite possible it is great that we've received a total of 14 pints (!) of ice cream as well as more chocolate than I can count as I'm trying to pack on some pre-chemo weight. However, as sweet as all my teeth are, I am having trouble keeping up and I hate to think of any of these treats going to waste! So although I'm not sure I ever thought I'd hear myself say/see myself write these words, and I would hate for this to be taken as non-appreciation, I think I must request that the sweet treats cease, at least for now, as we are truly overwhelmed by the amount of sugar that has been crossing our doorstep!

February 12, 2013

PGY-1 Shoutout

Many people think that being a doctor really adds a lot to this process - which is does - but not in the way one might expect. It's not my years of being an internist that are coming in handy, it's my year of being an intern that is the really turning out to be useful. It takes 4 years of medical school and at least 2 months of internship to do all the brilliant shit I've been doing!

- calling Kaiser to find out if they sent the slides to UCSF, then calling UCSF to find out if they got the slides from Kaiser (with Kaiser thinking that I was an administrator from UCSF and vice versa, I didn't lie, I just didn't volunteer the truth!), going straight to the pathologist to get the read on the slides, visiting with the pathology administrator to make sure she received the slides back from UCSF and was sending them to Dana Farber

- quickly and efficiently obtaining a copy of my medical records including CDs of all my scans

- contacting the referral dept directly to make sure they were faxing the referral authorization to the right place

- doing far more things in person (e.g. dropping by Kaiser to schedule an IR appointment) than by phone

- contacting departments to schedule appointments immediately after referrals are made rather than waiting for them to contact me

- rocket science, which was a big part of what I did as an intern as well as a big part of what I'm doing now, this shit is very medically complex!

- talking to social work early on to make sure that I can get into Laguna Honda when I'm ready for dispo

Wait, that one was a joke!

Even as I write this I'm eager to finish so that I can check "update blog" off my little list full of empty boxes.

Also a joke.

Sort of.

So, after not being able to convince oncologist #1 (O#1) to refer me to Stanford, and oncologist #2 (O#2) favoring the referral but not being able to place it since he is not my primary oncologist, I filed a grievance with Kaiser requesting the referral because a)this is rare b)this sucks c)nobody at Kaiser has ever treated it and d)the 2 opinions I've gotten at Kaiser have been about as opposite as can be. The review committee, which includes at least one physician, denied the request! They said that Kaiser has the expertise and they wanted to refer me to their "sarcoma group" which is obviously something of a joke because I've already seen the sarcoma "expert" at Kaiser. Fortunately, O#1 came through and spoke with the administrator and told them to approve my request since there isn't another sarcoma expert at Kaiser and I've gotten such different opinions. So I have an appt at Stanford in a week!

Not that I'll need it, because I spoke with the Stanford oncologist on the phone the other day and she recommends a year of chemo, and that I should start before I see her (?!?!?!). So, pretty easy to not start chemo before I see her (unless someone reading this has prescribing privileges in CA and is up for calling it in to the pharmacy for me?), but did mean that spring training no longer seems like an option (so we canceled, for the 2nd time). In case you're not keeping track, suggestions for treatment so far are:

1) watch and wait

2) surgery to remove all the mets, radiation, probably not chemo

3) chemo for a year, then surgery to take out anything that remains

28

Fortunately, all of these treatment recommendations are well validated in clinical trials and extremely well tolerated so I can't go wrong with any of them. It's almost like I have a bouquet with dozens of beautiful and different flowers and I just have to select the ones that are the prettiest!

Since only option #3 was suggested by someone who has ever seen a patient with mesenchymal cs unless she says something like "oh, I don't think chemo works, but it's fun so I think you should try it" I'll probably go with what she recommends. Not that I'm thrilled by the prospect of chemo, but it would be nice to have a plan so hopefully I'll have one in a week.

Besides, I've always wanted to be able to fit back into my bat mitzvah dress and I have long complained about the mucosa lining my oropharynx and am eager to see it go.

In my head the waiting room of the Stanford cancer center has comfy chairs and tazo tea and one of those keurig machines, and cucumber water, with some nice little snacks. I'll let you know.

February 13, 2013

MIL Shoutout

J and his mom just got matching tattoos! This is not J's first tattoo but it is his mom's. I am very impressed!

Mom, dad, you'll be pleased to know that I'm not expecting either one of you to follow suit.

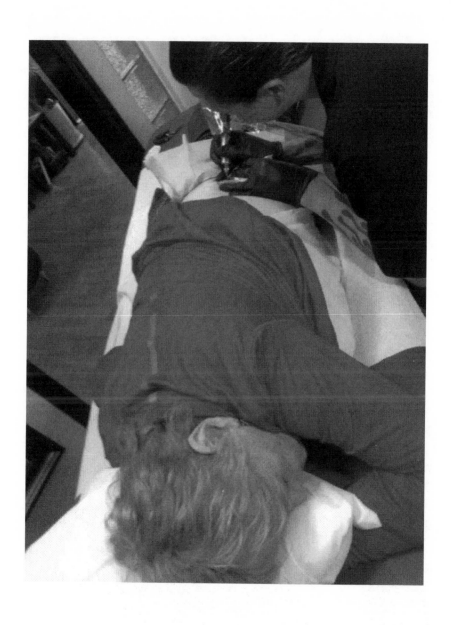

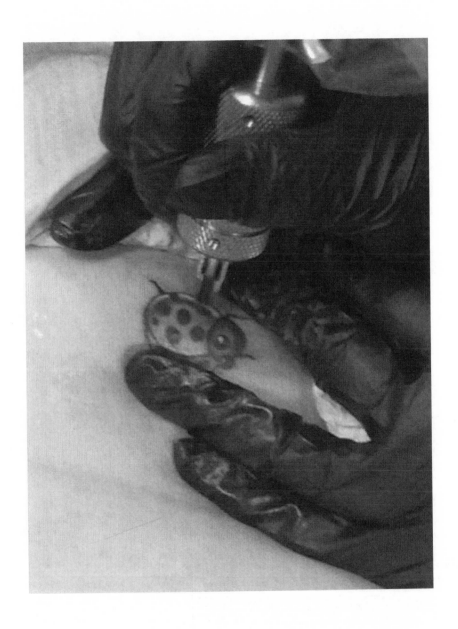

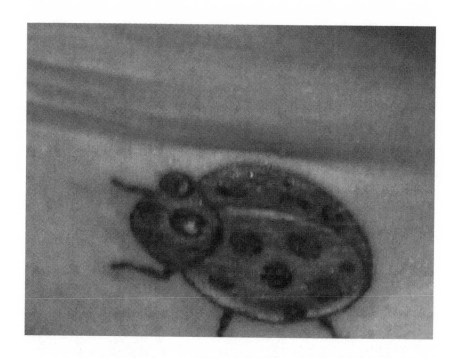

February 18, 2013

J's first day as an intern

J tracked down a CD of my bone scan! That's like 2nd
month of internship kind of work! We need it for appt
tomorrow at Stanford and went to the one place where you
can get them at Kaiser. The woman who does them was out
sick today and the person covering "left at 3:30" - which
must have been 3:30am since we were there before 3:30pm.
There was apparently nobody else who could help us. I had
an optho appt and it was close to 4pm which is basically

when everything closes, so I sent J to the radiology dept. and told him to try to get someone to burn a copy of the bone scan for us. While I was getting my eyes examined, he found someone who was incredibly helpful and got a copy of the scan! Go J! There were several non-helpful people mixed in there lest you think that Kaiser's all good, but I skipped those parts in this story for the sake of brevity and since the story is fascinating enough without those details.

In optho news, iritis flared when I tried to taper off the steroid drops (which I've been on since early Dec. btw). Also a little odd since it's mostly segmental and not involving all of my eye equally. So now I've officially got an unusual presentation of iritis - that nobody can connect to my other unusual presentation of something absurdly rare. There are case reports of orbital mesenchymal chondrosarcoma but from what I can tell those are all orbital tumors presenting with vision loss, proptosis, other mass-related effects, none of which I have. Another option is that this is all iatrogenic since 2 rounds of iritis resolved in less than a week without treatment and this episode was on its way to doing that until I went to optho because I needed to know if I really had recurrent iritis and was started on steroid drops. I'm off to see a Kaiser uveitis specialist on Monday and until then aggressive steroid drops.

For those of you who have really been paying attention, you may be wondering what happened to my valentine's day present of an ilium biopsy. I tallied all the votes and although the biopsy won the electoral college it lost the popular vote so I didn't do it. O#1 is the one who suggested, and ordered, it. But O#2 and ortho onc. didn't think it was necessary. And radiation oncology and O#3 (Stanford) were opposed to it. So, I "rescheduled" it for 3/1 but assume I'll cancel it.

I did meet with the radiation oncologist on Friday, she was of the "gee, chemo sounds really shitty" mindset and not surprisingly she suggests some radiation to the left ilium lesion rather than surgery (or chemo). But she also hasn't ever had a patient with mesenchymal cs. So really it's up to O#3 tomorrow to convince, or not convince, us that there's good reason to start chemo. If we're convinced, I've got a "chair" reserved for Monday afternoon and in another slick (if I do say so myself) move I got myself scheduled for a portacath this Thursday afternoon. I don't know that we'll be able to make a decision about chemo before then, unless O#3 is offering some sort of significant quality of life signing bonus if we agree to start while we're in her office, but again, it's more efficient to be on the schedule and have to reschedule.

In the meantime, J and I are still maintaining our "few things actually matter much" mindset which contributes to the consumption of large quantities of meat and other unhealthy entities, the occasional matinee (identity thief - cute), and the occasional, and opportune, ripping off the head of someone who is unaware of our situation (most recently the poor medical assistant who asked me about being several years behind on my cervical cancer screening - not that it matters, at all, but I'm actually not behind, it's just that I had Kaiser insurance before I went to medical school so they have it listed as "cervical cancer screen due March 1997.") I may have been a tad over-snarly in response to that question and I may or may not have said something like "I should be so lucky as to live long enough to die from cervical cancer."

35

Sorry medical assistant! Not your fault! I also believe in prevention!

It's actually amazing how frequently that idea comes in handy - I'm considering not flossing anymore.

I went to a beginner yoga class - I was hoping they would ask why we were there so I could say "well, I've got metastatic cancer and I know yoga will cure me" but they didn't ask. My favorite part was when I fell asleep, which happened more than once. Any stretch that one can fall asleep doing is a nice stretch! I'm thinking about going back but wearing noise-cancelling headphones so I don't have to listen to any of the spiritual bullshit; the stretching itself is great. Given the frequency with which women in yoga pants park their obama-sticker displaying prii (plural of prius) such that they block our driveway (one of several things that makes J wish he owned a shotgun, other things including people who don't use turn signals, everyone in the Berkeley Bowl parking lot), I pride myself on wearing the most yoga-inappropriate clothing I can find - I'm thinking overalls for the next class.

February 19, 2013

Officially this is terrible

Stanford oncologist says absolutely chemo, starting ASAP, Ewing's sarcoma inpatient regime of alternating cycles of vincristine, doxorubicin, cyclophosphamide and then ifosfamide and etoposide for a year. Restage after the first 3 months to see if things are getting smaller, if not, try some 2nd line agents. At the end, surgery to remove what's left, maybe some XRT.

Oh, and prognosis? Life expectancy of a year without chemo, maybe 2-4 years with chemo. Having trouble coming up with anything funny to say; hope that's not a longterm side effect of chemo.

February 21, 2013

Hang on a second

Well, even Kaiser thinks it's crazy that I've seen 3 oncologists with 3 different opinions (although only one has ever treated mesenchymal cs before), and O#1 offered to get me approved for a 4th opinion! So now I'm going to try for a telemedicine consult from Dana Farber. I get all my records and scans to the sarcoma expert there and he provides a written opinion. I'm assuming he'll still suggest chemo (and by assuming I mean that I had a portacath placed yesterday and I chopped off all my hair today) but it could be a different regimen. So, for now, chemo is off for Monday morning and I'm scheduled for the following Monday morning. Now I just need to get my records to DF ASAP! In many ways I just wanted to get going with this, but I would feel better if one other person who has treated this confirmed the treatment plan before I start down this path.

I decided that even if I'm not doing chemo I won't want to be in the hospital recovering from a thoracotomy with long hair, so I went ahead with the haircut today. I'm not even that traumatized.

And for those of you thinking that "finally, the selfishness ends, an opportunity for her to think about someone else for a minute" - no such luck - turns out my hair was too layered to be donated to make a wig for some kid with cancer.

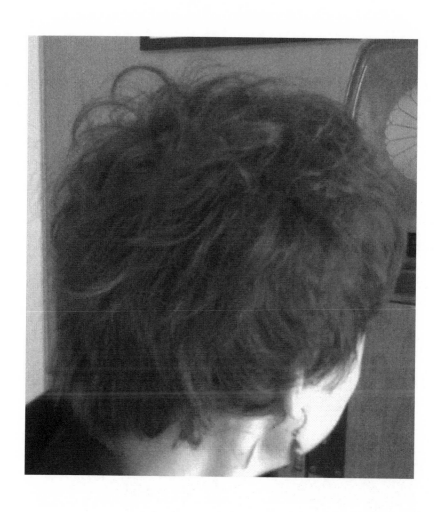

February 22, 2013

Salazon Chocolate

Will the person who sent us the salazon chocolate please stand up? We'd love to thank him/her/them but we're not sure who sent it!

February 23, 2013

Most practical gift so far?

Bedazzled emesis basin! Thanks CBSnJCTH!

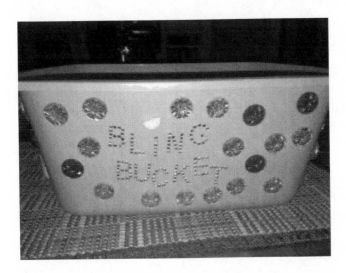

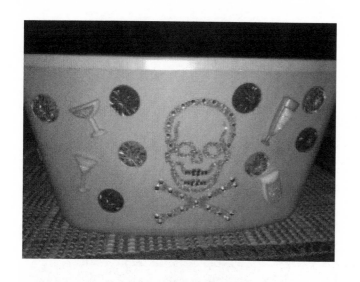

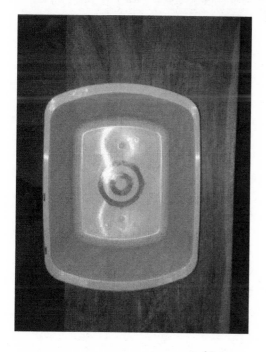

February 28, 2013

What a difference

another oncologist makes.

Not to pick favorites or anything, but if there is an annual Stanford Cancer Center/Dana Farber softball game I am totally rooting for Dana Farber. We got the formal opinion from them last night, in the form of the oncologist (Dana Farber guy, DFG) calling us at 10:30 pm (his time) to spend 90 minutes on the phone with us discussing my case. The most important thing he did was leave us with the sense that there's certainly no guarantee that the prognosis is as dire, or precise, as Stanford lady (SL) suggested. The numbers he quoted are that based on the small number of small case series 20-60% of patients with mes. cs are alive at 10 years. Right now that sounds not too different from him telling me that I'll be living in a nursing home playing pinochle 50 years from now. Well, at least in comparison to SL to whom I thought I should send a post-appointment text message that I made it back to the car without dropping dead from cancer. We're not under any illusions about how shitty this all could be, but DF gave us some hope which had been surgically removed from our bodies, mixed with dogshit, and flushed down the toilet at Stanford. I should also point out that they had no cucumber water, tazo tea, keurig, or snacks and in addition to being felt-up by an oncology fellow doing a totally unnecessary lymph node exam (I know, I know, they've got to learn, blah, blah, blah) we had to have our conversation about my imminent death in an exam room with the fellow crouched in the corner. Really, the Stanford Cancer Center doesn't have an office where patients can receive their expensive second opinions while actually facing their doctor? I bet DF has kouign-amann and a barista pulling espresso shots in their waiting room.

DFG's recommendation isn't that different but he sure made everything sound different - 2 3-week cycles of chemo, both vincristine, doxorubicin, and cyclophosphamide, then re-stage and go from there. Perhaps more chemo, perhaps different chemo, perhaps surgery plus a hint of radiation. He didn't think that it was critical that I start immediately, but he recognized the psychological aspect of wanting to feel something is being done. He also said it's better to do chemo when you're feeling healthy than waiting until you're symptomatic from your cancer. So, I start on Monday, wish me luck!

It's hard to explain how much better we felt after talking to DFG last night. Perhaps it can best be summed up by J's post-call exclamation "Great, so now we can be done with everything being about you all the time! Now you can start taking care of me!" Perhaps slightly less telling is that the conversation made me wish that I was doing the kind of clinical medicine that would afford me the opportunity to have that type of substantial relationship with patients/families in the hope that I would provide the kind of care for them that DFG gave us.

Bedazzled emesis basin, here comes me!

February 28, 2013

Cancer Zinger #2

And, the award for the best set-up goes to W, a VA employee who called me to tell me that my my transportation pass was ready and I would need to pick it up in person. When I told her that I was out on medical leave and wouldn't be picking it up anytime soon she actually said "Oh, that doesn't sound good, after all the time I spent doing this paperwork and now you can't even use the pass…" I quickly glanced at the heavens to thank Jesus for delivering this set-up to me on a platinum platter, giddy with excitement about what was about to happen, and interrupted her to say "I was just diagnosed with metastatic cancer and have been told I may be dead in a year, so I apologize for whatever inconvenience the paperwork may have caused you but that pales in comparison to what I'm dealing with so you'll have to understand why I do not care." She sort of apologized and then hung-up.

It may never get any better than that.

But one can hope.

March 3, 2013

Chemo Countdown!

Ready!

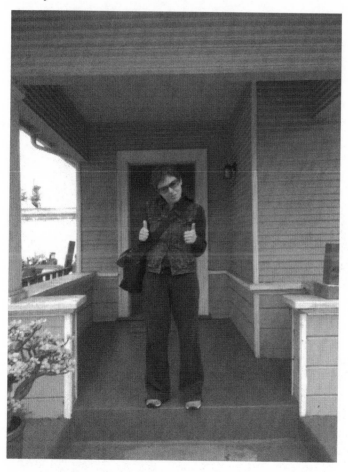

Set!

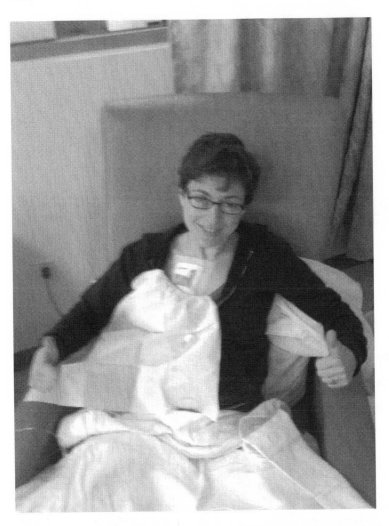

Go!

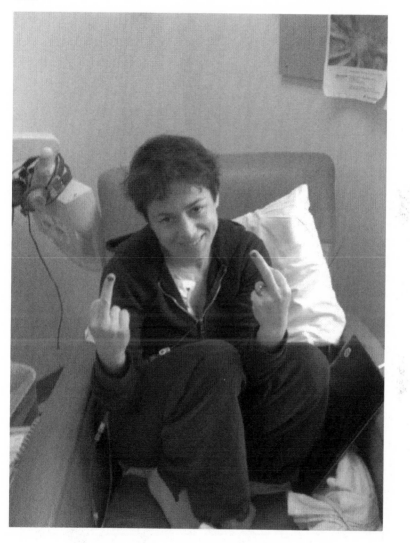

March 4, 2013

Contest!

If anyone is so inclined and familiar with this sort of thing and wants to suggest a different tumblr format I'm all ears! There are a zillion options and I just want something basic, with the newest posts at the top, ideally with the date as something separate from the title. I'm even willing to pay for one. I have not had the patience to scroll through all the options but if there is someone out there for whom this is an easy and fun task please feel free to make some suggestions! In return, if your format is selected, you will win my great appreciation, you will have bragging rights and a sense of ownership and pride every time you look at the blog, and I will consider sending you all of my leftover narcotics and other controlled substances when this is over - pending evaluation of your addiction potential.

March 4, 2013

Round 1

Another day, more chemo, this is it for 3 weeks. There were two other young people in there today - I gave one of them the "maybe we should try to get pediatric oncologists so we don't feel like the most tragic cases sitting in the waiting room" nod. I do feel a very strong desire to wear a t-shirt that says "nope, not breast cancer!" Although I think there's an separate oncology suite reserved for the breast cancer patients

48

where everything (walls, chairs, medical equipment) is pink and sponsored by the Susan G. Komen foundation.

They tell me to expect to feel shitty through the weekend, then things should start picking up. I mostly slept after getting home yesterday - sleep for 3 hours, up for an hour or two, repeat. Since they had slightly overdosed me on dexamethasone that was really the opposite of what was supposed to have happened. Some mild nausea, pleased to say no vomiting. The meds are supposed to hold me well through tomorrow, then might be a little rougher. I haven't had much of an appetite but am trying to eat some stuff. Not much seems appealing, unfortunately. They told me to focus on liquids and not worry about eating solids if I'm not up for it this week.

Today I actually went for a little walk! J was worried about me and insisted I only walk around the block, and repeat if necessary, but not go further away. I was in my 3rd lap wondering if people were thinking I was casing their place when I noticed a car following me. I was in the process of texting J to tell him perhaps this wasn't the best neighborhood for walking around the block repeatedly while wearing sunglasses, a baseball cap, and a hooded sweatshirt, when I realized that J was the one following me. He's a little worried about me. He thinks I'm not a very good patient. I disagree somewhat, I think I'm an ok patient. I'm certainly not planning on my "time-off" during chemo to be when I finally train for that triathlon or learn Spanish. At this point my main goal is to rotate my sitting and lying spots so I don't get sick of any of them too quickly.

I hope I'll have more entertaining things to say in the future and this won't just be a daily log of my sleeping, eating, and bowel habits. No way Dr. Oz is gonna sponsor me if that's all I come up with.

March 6, 2013

There will be edema

The original title of the Daniel Day-Lewis movie that was going to be about a quest for wealth resulting in the accumulation of fluid in his legs, but apparently that wasn't captivating enough for Hollywood.

I wasn't prepared for 10lb of post-chemo water-weight. Since my heart and kidneys are still functioning I'm assuming this is not a harbinger of impending heart or kidney failure. Also, it's better today than yesterday which is all I'm asking for at this point. As it turns out, J loves me extra-squishy so he's thrilled by this development.

Suffered a slight setback today when I foolishly thought I was in a post-ondansetron state - turns out it still serves a purpose! I have never been so appreciative of Big Pharma before, really, they are just wonderful and they should just keep doing exactly what they are doing! Just a few hours of nausea, nothing big, rescued by some ginger-ale and Angry Bird graham crackers. Overall I've been doing quite well. I even ate some real food yesterday and went for a walk. Hoping to get out for a walk today too.

Seriously, that is all I have to report. The entertaining part of this blog may now be over.

March 13, 2013

Wait a minute!

I was prepared for the nausea (which was far less bad than expected, I pray to the god I don't believe in that it stays that way), I was prepared for the fatigue, I was prepared for the hair loss (well, actually, that hasn't happened yet and I'm definitely not prepared for it b/c I know once that happens everyone will realize I'm sick whereas now they just think I'm mildly grumpy, which wasn't so different from before, though now has the distinct, inevitable, advantage that some day, some where, some poor suckers is gonna say "smile, it can't be that bad" and I'm gonna get to say "oh really, how does this sound...") but for some reason I just decided that now, 11 days after my first chemo, was a good time to read about the food I'm not supposed to eat, and I am not on board with that shit! No raw milk cheese? A cheesemaker friend of the family in Connecticut just sent us a few pounds of amazing stuff. No honey? For the first week post-chemo my most delicious meal was a smoothie, made by J, with yogurt, frozen berries, banana, and a touch of honey. And no, there wasn't any of that wheatgrass crap in there, or protein powder, or anything else that would make it seem like something other than just fat and sugar peeking out from behind the skirt of a fake piece of fruit. Some debate as to whether the smoothie was inherently delicious or whether I've just discovered why yogurt wasn't invented as nonfat. No sushi? Ok, actually, chemo and sushi never seemed like a good combo to me so I'm not that freaked out or surprised about missing it. Lox? Right, like this is the point in my life when I'm going to stop eating smoked fish. Bacon, sausage, hot dogs? With baseball season around the corner? What am I going to eat at the ballpark? Hummus platter? Sidewalk vendors? Surely that doesn't include taco trucks since they are not actually located on a sidewalk? And the icing on the cake, unpasteurized beer? The stuff that my husband makes gallons of every week? The only activity that keeps him sane? The brewing of beer is by far one of the most positive things that goes on in our house these days, and I'm not supposed to drink any of it? I suspect that means I'm also not supposed to sleep in the same room where the yeast is bubbling away?

On the plus side, I have worried that being one of the 30-90 new cases of mesenchymal cs in the US is not enough for a case report (which, it's not); if I get a weird disseminated yeast infection from sleeping in the same room as brewers yeast that would probably bump me up.

So, yeah, the first round of chemo was far, far more tolerable than I imagined it might be. I realize they'll only get worse but at least one round is done and after spending last week mostly in bed, sleeping, mildly nauseated, not eating a lot, I was up and walking around by Friday and since then have had a pretty normal appetite and have gotten out at least a little bit most days. But if I'm really not supposed to eat any of that stuff, and if I'm supposed to follow essentially the same diet as a pregnant woman, but not be pregnant, and not have any kids, and have had 3 miscarriages, and never be able to have any kids cause chemo is going to make my reproductive system even less functional than it already is, well, I don't know if I'm ready to do that for a year.

But, otherwise, I've been feeling pretty good. Some people have been worried I wasn't writing because I wasn't feeling well but I guess it was closer to the opposite of that.

March 14, 2013

Nothing to do with cancer

For those of you paying attention, J loves brewing beer. The only thing he loves almost as much as brewing beer is beer brewing equipment. His new brew kettle arrived today. It holds 10 gallons and has a spigot. We thought it was coolly made in the US (in a modern, 2010's, locavore sort of way, not an old-fashioned, 1970's, jingoistic sort of way) - but it was made in China. J wasn't home when it arrived and he asked me to send him a photo of it, so I did, and I'm posting them below because sometimes it's nice to not talk about cancer.

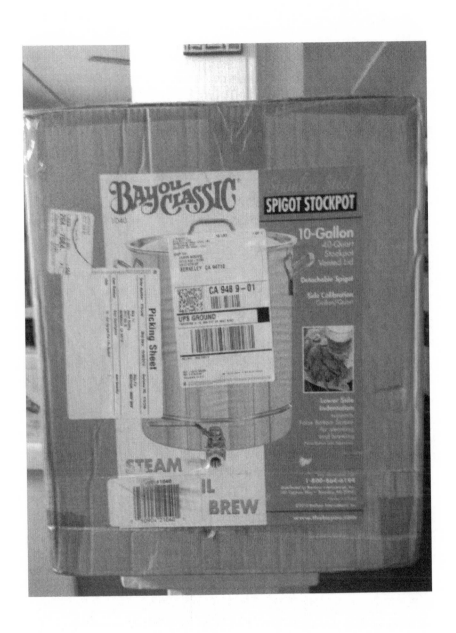

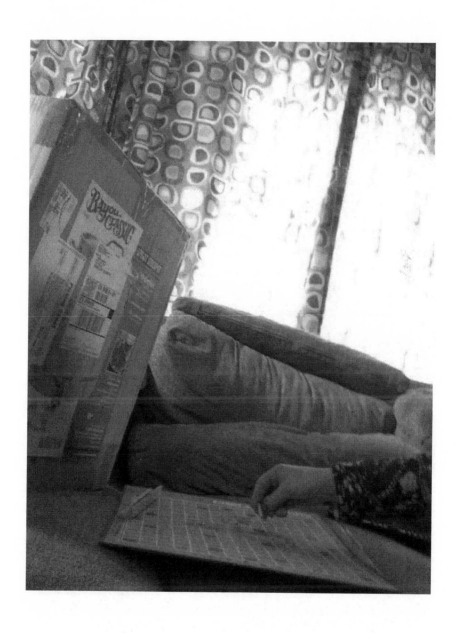

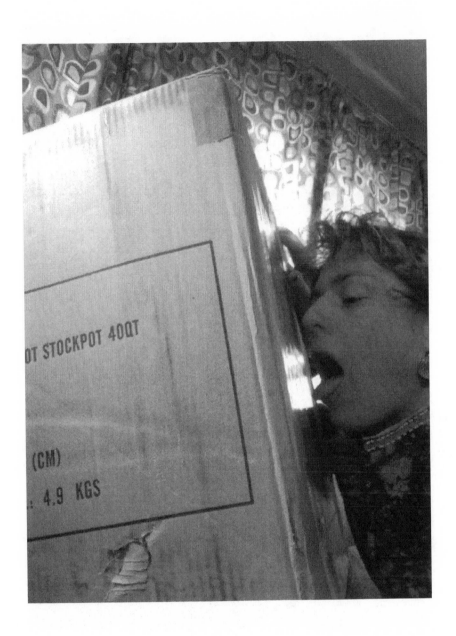

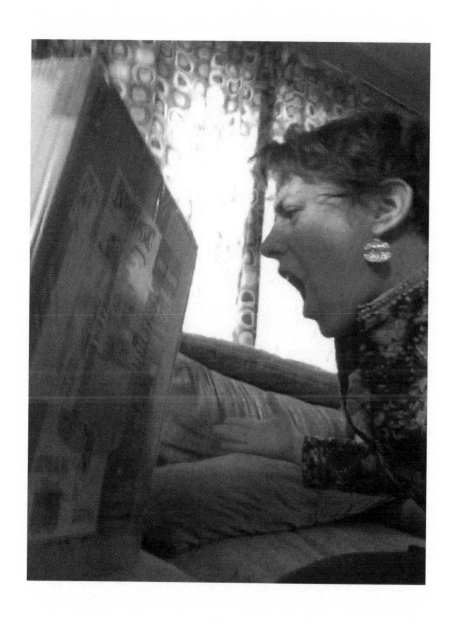

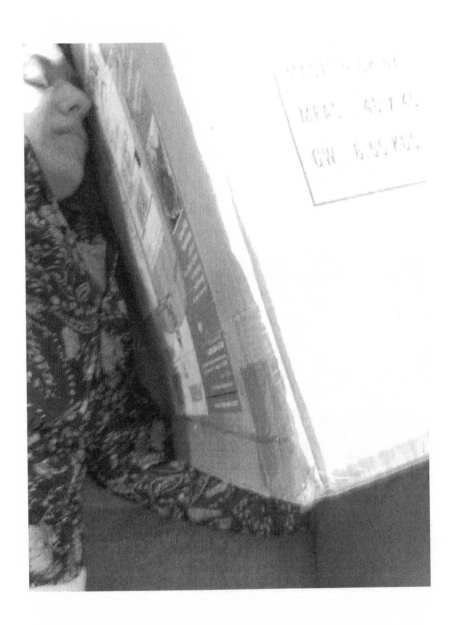

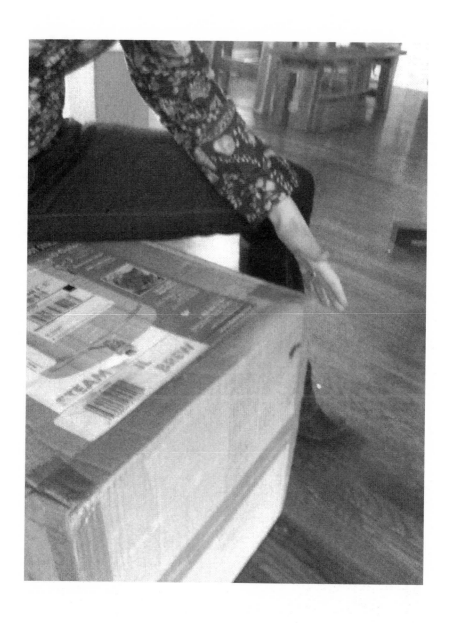

March 18, 2013

Hair starting to come out!

Ack!

Still looks totally normal but shedding is moderately distressing. Considering preemptive buzzcut.

March 19, 2013

Clipping Day!

un

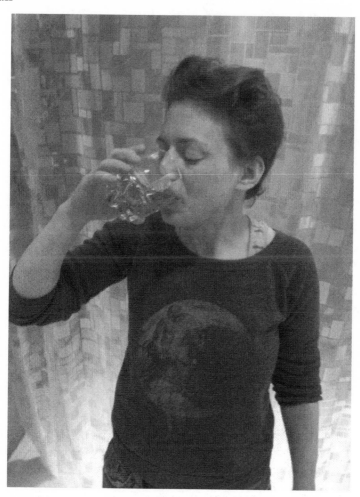

deux

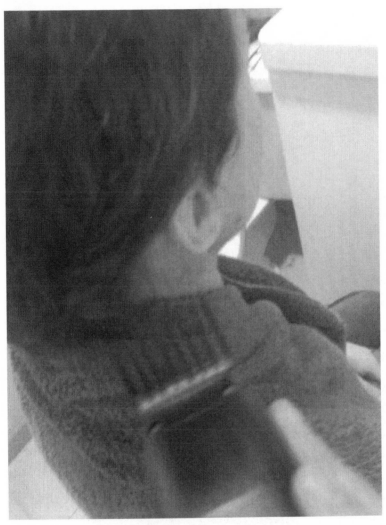

trois

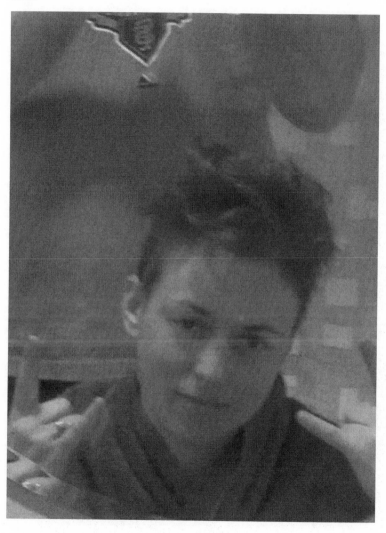

quatre

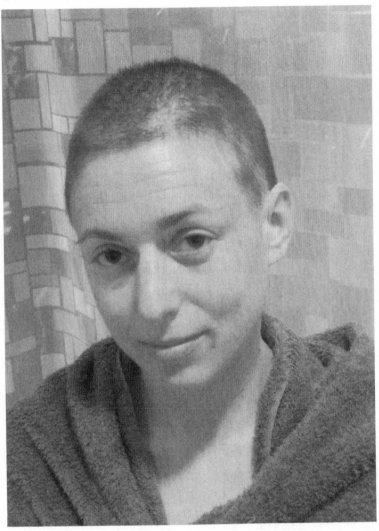

cinq

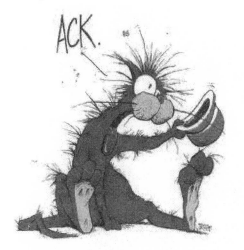

J's turn

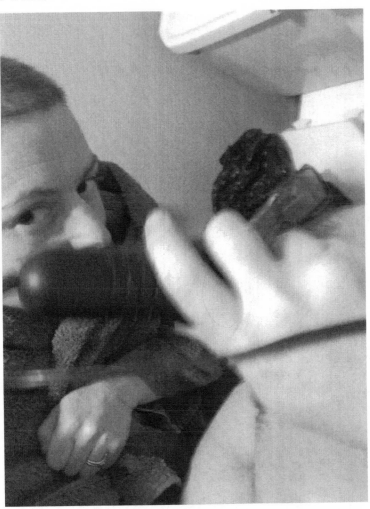

March 20, 2013

Shopping with cancer

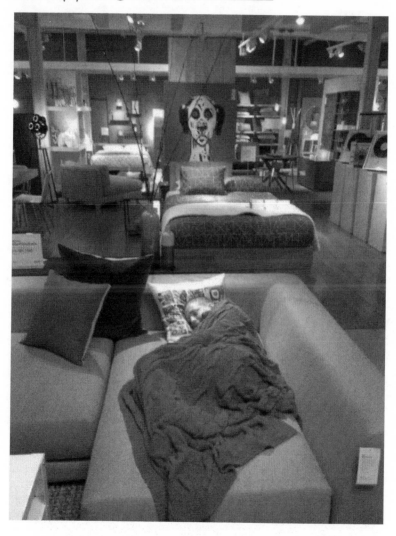

Actually, I was just testing out the couch, but I figure I can do whatever the hell I want with this new do.

March 21, 2013

For those of you who have been wondering

what the top of my head looks like

here you go!

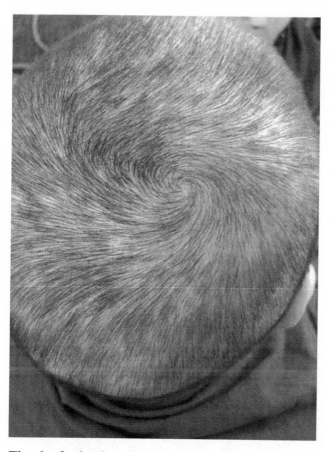

Thanks for having that c-section, mom!

Down to a 1 on the clippers, next stop, bald!

March 23, 2013

Living life to the fullest the day before chemo

J: How many Bob Dylan songs do you know?

Me: Do I know? I don't know.

J: Does one know?

Me: I don't know.

J: A lot.

Me: Was that whole thing just a rhetorical question?

J: Yes.

Me: I'd like that time back.

J: Yeah, we should probably be more careful.

March 25, 2013

Blech!

On the "chemo is fun" scale, this round is ranking lower than last round, so far. Although, in fairness (to the cyclophosphamide, vincristine, and doxorubicin), the the nausea is still controlled enough such that I have not needed to vomit (yay!). But since arriving home at 4pm yesterday I have been in bed until just now - and now I'm on the couch which some might argue is not that different than being in bed. I'm a tad nervous about getting more today although once I'm there I figure they can protect me from most things. Big Pharma don't fail me now!

AC can attest to the lengths to which I will go to abate nausea. Several years ago, we were sea kayaking in SE Alaska and despite his contention that only children get motion sick, I felt quite ill when we were out in the open in the moderately (by kayak standards) rough waves. I kayaked with what can only be described as the speed, and skill, of an olympic kayaker to the nearest piece of land, which turned out to be essentially a large rock. Like a parent lifting an 18-wheeler to remove his/her child trapped beneath, I covered what must have been 5 (nautical) miles in a mere 20 minutes determined to scale whatever I needed to scale to get myself and the kayak on to solid land. Fortunately, climbing equipment was not necessary, and I was able to get out onto that magical "island." Also fortunately, AC kindly decided to follow me so I didn't end up getting stranded. And after a brief respite, I was able to continue on, un-ill. But I haven't gone sea kayaking since.

Oh, and where is my rock in the middle of the sea now?

Ah, the ondansetron, it's been 8 hours since my last one, taking it now. All good!

March 26, 2013

And on the third day

after chemo

God invented pozole.

My goodness that pozole J just brought me was delicious. Obviously my nausea is somewhat improved. I even showered, got "dressed" (loosely defined these days and not too different from what I sleep in), and went for a little walk today! I anticipate a dip in how I'm feeling tomorrow as the stronger anti-emetic wears off but I'm appreciating the feeling ok-ish as it exists currently.

April 4, 2013

I figured it out

There is a strong correlation between kaiser visits and blog posts because in the absence of interacting with the medical system this whole experience is not really that absurd or humorous. At the beginning I had tons of visits, thus tons of blog posts - more recently, all I've had are chemo visits (which are actually less absurd and humorous than one might think). I just did the math, because, I've got that kind of time, and nearly 60% of all blog posts occurred either the day of or the day after some sort of medical appointment/test/procedure. I didn't even exclude ones for which I was sedated!

So, in keeping with tradition, I write today because I went to Kaiser today! I figured with the whole "terrible cancer diagnosis" thing it might be a good idea for me to talk to a therapist. So I made an appt to see one at Kaiser. I quickly found out that Kaiser doesn't do individual therapy - at all! Even the psychologist didn't think that I was a great candidate for group therapy (although I can see how that would make me quite prolific, blog-wise). But no, even when the provider doesn't think that Kaiser offers what is indicated, Kaiser won't cover outside care - amazing! Before I get further into this, I will say that I believe the person I saw genuinely wants to help me and was certainly trying her best and I don't think she's an idiot. She wants to see me 3-4 times to help determine what would be helpful for me - and I gather that is not something that she offers most/many people.

That being said…

I will go at least once more, mostly to see what else she comes up with, because her first suggestions were nothing short of hilarious. She does not think that psychoanalysis would be helpful since it is too slow-going and abstract and she thinks some specific tools would be most helpful. A good deal of our first visit was spent with her reading excerpts to me from the wikipedia page on Ericksonian Hypnosis - something she thinks would be very useful for me (of course I'll have to pay out of pocket to go see someone outside Kaiser to get it). Another suggestion had something to do with telling "spiritual stories of healing," which, even though I realize this blog would technically count as one of those, if anybody refers to this as either spiritual or a healing story I'm going to vomit (and it won't have anything to do with chemo). She briefly mentioned alternative therapy and I was eager to ask her if she thought that yoga would have the side benefit of curing my cancer but I decided not to go there. She also recommended a women's cancer center that focuses on low-income women of color, although she acknowledged that I may not be their target audience. And finally, she provided me with the brochure for a cancer support group; although it is in Walnut Creek, the drumming circle they offered reassured me that they are still part of the Bay Area.

So, in brief, options at Kaiser for mental health care include: drugs, group activities (with and without drums, some with beads and crystals), and that's about it.

Color me impressed.

Look, I know lots of different things are helpful for lots of different people, and it's wonderful that people find things that work for them. But I've decided that I'm going to die the way that I've lived and that is, among other things, as a skeptic. And I would rather go out unpleasantly than go out as a very comfortable, yet completely different person, who believes that hypnosis and juicing saved me.

I've decided to aim low and just hope that people remember me as consistent.

April 16, 2013

Good News!

The chemo is doing something - I had the repeat PET scan and there are no new lesions, the existing lesions are not larger, and there is reduced metabolic activity in all 4 lesions. While all 4 are the same size, it just seems good that they are somewhat less active. So it seems that the chemo is doing something and is worth continuing. The plan is for another two cycles (the first of which started this Monday) and then repeat PET. As long as there continues to be some type of improvement, and I'm tolerating the chemo, this will go on for a bit (6 months? 1 year? Not clear to me). If there is no more improvement or I'm not tolerating the regimen it's likely I'll switch to another regimen for 2 cycles and continue that for a bit if it's working. If chemo isn't working and/or is sucking, then perhaps some surgery/xrt is in my future. But at least for now I'm on the chemo train for a while. So we're stocking up on ondansetron, smoothie ingredients, and ginger ale. You might think sunblock but I've been going bald, hatless, and sunblockless because I think it would be hilarious if I got skin cancer while doing chemo. Still trying to work all the funny angles here.

April 20, 2013

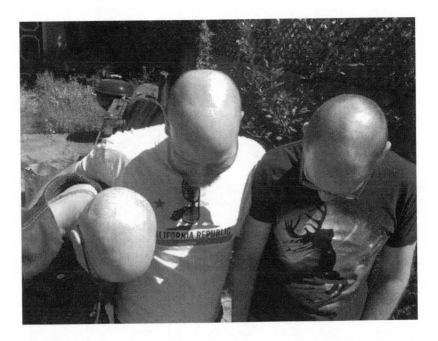

Solidarity

April 24, 2013

Food Perversions

I'm still doing fairly well with the chemo, but man is it eating
(ha!) away at my eating options. The other day I called 4

bakeries to see what kind of scones they had in an attempt to find one that seemed appealing since a scone was just about the only thing I could think of that sounded good to eat.

Some of you might think that I have always been the kind of person to call a bakery to ask about their scone selection but that's really not the case! Sadly, all of the varieties sounded crappy and J found me stomping around the house muttering to myself wondering why anyone would add chocolate to a scone - he grabbed me by the shoulders and told me to pull it together, while he laughed at me - which was actually quite effective.

It seems like every day a new food item falls victim to being associated with nausea. Certainly anything I eat the week of chemo ends up on my shit list (the shit list consists of foods that seem less appealing to eat than does a pile of shit). But now there is a component of randomness by which any food may at any point end up on the shit list. And since nothing seems to come off the shit list, I worry that I will be left with little as this progresses.

Shit list so far:
meat (red, white, other)
seafood
avocado (really tragic since, oddly, for a while cucumber and avocado sushi was one of my main post-chemo meals)
Vietnamese, Korean, and Thai food

I spend a fair amount of time trying to come up with foods that sound appealing to eat. Occasionally, a random association will reveal a new option. For instance, walking past a gentleman of middle-eastern descent made me crave hummus. Passing by a store that sold "flotation devices" brought the remarkable rootbeer float into my every day (currently wondering if it's an appropriate breakfast item, also had a dream about one last night - in which it was served with raspberry ice cream and I had to protest). Other items that are still good to go include Indian food (living 2 blocks from Viks has been wonderful, though I fear Indian food will eventually go the way of its Asian brethren), yogurt, fruit - on a real berries and citrus kick right now, eggs, cereal, oatmeal, and, of course, scones, as long as they don't contain chocolate.

May 4, 2013

"I've seen worse"

Those are the sort of comforting words I hear from my oncologist when he evaluates how I've been doing with the chemo.
Actually, I'm fine with that. I'm happy to be told I'm handling chemo fairly well, and I find his slightly less than touchy-feely attitude to be funny.
Other things I think are funny:
1. http://www.youtube.com/watch?feature=player_embedded&v=VGZcerOhCuo
Is it just me or is this absurd? I spent the whole commercial thinking that the health worker was doing all this travel and they were sending all those resources there to provide medical care. Reminded me of the character in The League who was ""DJ-ing in Haiti for the villagers." Heartbeats

don't make for a very interesting rhythm anyway, do they? It would have been better if the kids had irregular heartbeats and then instead of figuring out what was wrong with them they just made a really funky song out of their arrhythmias.
2. When we find parkng right out front some place we are going and there is money in the meter and J says "oh man, we are soooo lucky." I like to say that we do our luck the way we do our finances, penny lucky, pound unlucky.
3. This hat
http://www.tlcdirect.org/Embroidered-Cotton-Denim-Bucket.html?did=64
and the text accompanying another hat they sell "Of course, no hat will look good if you lack eyebrows. Our Eazy Brow Eye Brow Stencil solves this problem…"
Way to try to make money while insulting someone who already feels fairly shitty about how s(he) looks.
4. This billboard

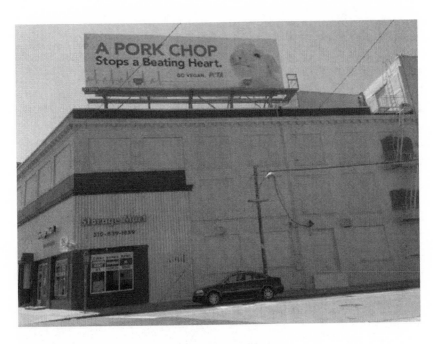

More chemo Monday and Tuesday...

May 5, 2013

New and improved!

Thanks to AC's efforts, the blog is (IMHO, as the kids say) better! You'll note that the main page is no longer blank, the entries appear in reverse chronological order with the newest ones on the top, and there is a "table of contents" on the right side of the page. Also, if you hover over the end of the post the date shows up so I no longer have to include it in the title AND you can add comments!

As promised, AC gets any controlled substances that I have leftover at the end of all this.

May 8, 2013

Cross purposes

J loves it when I'm all edematous from chemo - he prefers me soft and blobby.

And he laughs at my "perfectly spherical" head.

Is this considered supportive?

He does rub my puffy feet so I think that counts.

May 13, 2013

Coming out from under

Fairly blechy round. Not sure if this is what is meant by the effects being cumulative or if it was the extra anti-emetics that kept me more bed-oriented than usual. I seem to be turning a corner today, but as the 14 episodes of Entourage I watched yesterday can attest to, I am less functional than I

81

have been at this point in rounds past. The biggest issue is that this has pushed me a week back in my quest to be a volunteer dog walker at the animal shelter. I haven't found some sort of new purpose in life, but the animal shelter is about 3 blocks away and when I am up for walking I go right by it so I figure I can walk a dog at the same time and at least do something mildly useful with my time (see "Entourage," above). Although I'm only familiar with the dog walking requirements, I'm fairly certain that it's more challenging to become a dog walker than it is to adopt a child. I know you think I'm exaggerating for the sake of humor, but I'm really not! First I had to complete an application, then I had to attend a 2 hour orientation filled with so much earnest good-heartedness that I regretted not bringing some anti-emetics with me. The orientation was going well until I accidentally hit the volume button on my phone and everyone in the room heard Blanco's at-bat. I was really looking forward to asking them why they vaccinate the dogs and cats, since that's what makes them autistic, but since I had already established myself as a rogue volunteer I was worried about getting kicked-out. The next step is to attend a 90 minute dog-walking class, and I was going to go on Saturday but I felt too crappy so now I have to wait until next week! And the class is not the last step! After the class, I will be assigned a "mentor" who will accompany me on several walks to make sure that I'm ready to walk a dog on my own.

Seriously, I could not make this shit up.

Speaking of absurd shit I cannot make up. Our oddish neighbor (who J accurately describes as being stuck in 1983) called me over when I was leaving the house and we had the following conversation.

N: Is everything OK, Rachel?

Me: Yes.

N: It's just that a few of the neighbors have been talking, and we're not sure if the new hairdo is to help out kids with cancer or something.

Me: No. I have bone cancer; I'm getting chemotherapy.

N: Oh no! That's terrible! We are all here for you should you need anything.

<awkard embrace>

N: So, what do you think of my thumb? I think I jammed it the other night.

May 18, 2013

Hair today.

A number of you have contacted me to let me know that you haven't been able to sleep as you are wondering about the status of my hair. I apologize for the sleepless nights I may have caused. At long last, the update for which you have been waiting.

I've learned a lot of things about the hair on the top of my head. For one thing, it takes up a lot of space! Now that I don't have it, I've had to adjust my baseball cap several sizes (I tried it unadjusted, but then J said "nothing says cancer like a bald woman in an oversized baseball cap.") Furthermore, it really keeps your head warm! Since I mostly refuse to wear a hat because I hate to look like I'm trying to hide my baldness, I spend a lot of time being really cold. Coincidentally, I've also noticed that it seems like a lot of heat comes out of it! I say this because when I get into bed I have to flip my pillow over after a few minutes because the part of the pillow previously responsible for holding my head has literally burst into flames.

Not all of my hair fell out and I was feeling like the guys who stayed behind were just being supportive. You know, sort of a "I really found out who my friends were when I got cancer and started chemotherapy and that little patch of hair on the upper right part of my head stuck with me through the whole thing" kind of thing. But then J pointed out that it was really patchy and was putting me somewhat at the mercy of the chemo and if I really wanted to "own" the baldness we should shave the head.

So we did that yesterday.

But then I found out that J found my prickly little head "annoying" when he snuggled up against it. And he made a comment about my head being a landing pad for the world's smallest helicopter. And then I saw this.

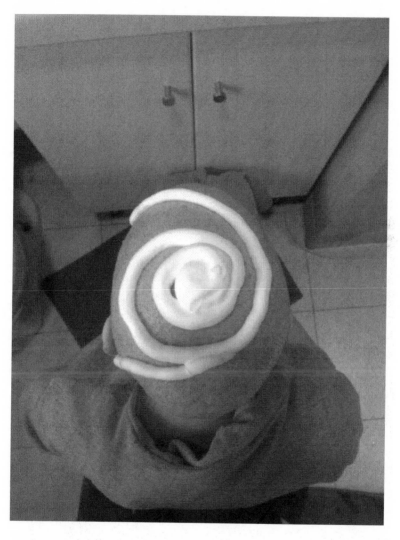

So now I'm not sure if this was all about a husband doing an incredibly sweet, loving, thing for his wife or a husband

having fun at his wife's expense and having soft, smooth area to rest his chin?
It is really soft and smooth though.

May 20, 2013

Operation Dog Walk, continued

Yesterday I attended a 90 minute "dog walking class" as the third step of my plan to become a volunteer dog walker at the animal shelter.

This is the dog with which I worked.

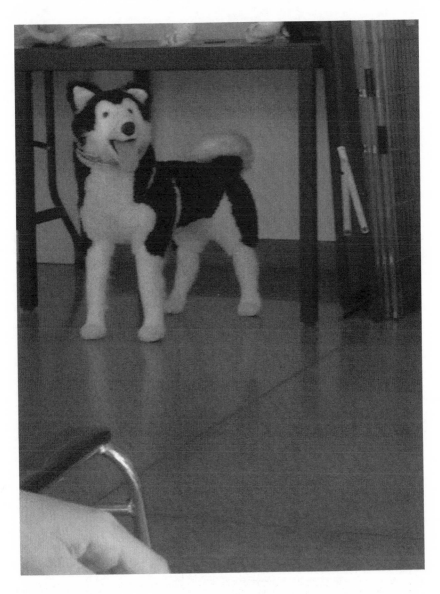

She didn't bite.

Or bark.

Or move.

Just to be clear, I attended a 90 minute "dog walking" class and no live dogs were present. Even when I walked in and noticed that there were 3 different-sized stuffed dogs, and I nearly choked on my own laughter, I assumed that we would practice (?!?I) something on these dogs *and then actually walk a dog*! But no, we spent the class *talking* about walking dogs. I think we could have done it in fewer than 90 minutes but half the class was under the age of 12 and they took us off topic on several occasions. One girl volunteered that she was not scared of pit bulls because her friend has a pit bull named Pearl who is very sweet. I considered telling her that that's a really cute story but isn't actually relevant. I was impressed with the girl in front of me who asked some very on-point questions, but for the most part I thought the kids didn't do a great job of restricting their questions to topics of interest to the class as a whole. It reminded me of the large intro public health classes I took in which people straight out of college would ask, in a room of 300 students, questions like "can I take the midterm on a different day because it conflicts with a conference I have to attend?"

So, the dog walking saga continues. The next step is to be assigned a mentor and arrange a time to walk a dog with him/her. I should have confirmed that the dog we will be walking will be real.

May 27, 2013

Ok, here's the situation

The good news is that the PET scan I just had showed further reduced metabolic activity and no new mets. All 4 lesions are still there, and they are the same size, but at least the chemo seems to be doing something. So the plan is to do 2 more rounds of this chemo which will pretty much get me to the max dose of doxorubicin because of the risk of cardiac toxicity with additional doses. Then we'll do another PET scan, take a break for a few weeks, and repeat the PET. Depending on what has happened off treatment we'll decide if we are going to watch and wait, do more (different) chemo, surgery, and/or radiation. The waiting around part won't be fun but I am looking forward to a break from chemo! It does mean that I will probably have to stop claiming that pie is an appropriate dinner but I'm not going to broach that conversation with myself until after these next two rounds.

So, off to chemo tomorrow!

May 27, 2013

Speaking of awesome things that have happened to me...

Here I am with Barry Zito at the baseball game yesterday! Thank you GC for making me the physician representative for The Veterans Health Research Institute (http://www.ncire.org/) as part of the Giant's Memorial Day on-field salute to veterans and active military!

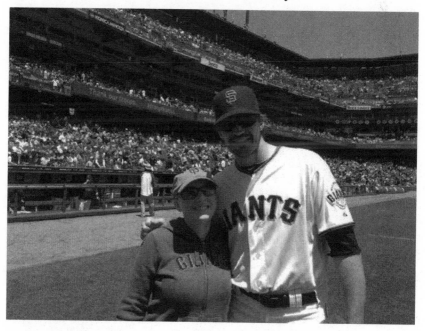

It was a little annoying that Zito insisted on standing on a stool just so that it would appear that he towers over me.

June 3, 2013

Two steps forward

One small step back.

Felt ill on this day 8, drank some water and vomited so decided to go in. This is my first chemo emesis! I do not understand how people managed/manage chemo when it was/is emesis-centric. That is some insane strength. I threw up some water and was ready to dig out my portacath with a plastic straw and donate it to a homeless shelter. Since I also vomited when I was waiting to check-in (may blessings rain down on the clerk who got me an emesis thing in time and then brought me a cool wet cloth) they gave me another round of anti-emetics. My vitals weren't bad and my labs are fine. My big concern is that now that I've vomited water I may never drink water again. They'll say "wow, she beat her cancer but it was so sad when she died from dehydration because she refused to drink water." I'm anemic but no more than I was a week ago (my hemoglobin was around 12 pre-chemo and is now around 8). But I'm feeling symptomatic and vasovagally - you should see me walk up a flight of stairs! And on more than one occasion only the muttering of the phrase "don't pass out" seems to have kept me from passing out on the commode. So, I'm going back tomorrow for a transfusion. I feel like I'm really not so anemic that I should need one, but since I don't feel great and I suspect I will feel pretty perky post-blood it seems worth doing. Turns out I'm a universal recipient (AB) and J is a universal donor (O) which we either didn't know or didn't remember. We are now working on our soon-to-be bestselling book "Snuggle For Your Blood Type."

The worst part is that I was going to have my first 2-hour dog-walking mentor session tomorrow morning but now I can't do it because of the transfusion!!!

Curses, foiled again!

June 5, 2013

True blood

Got my 2 units of PRBCs yesterday, came home and went for a little walk, ate a mess of pasta, cleaned up the kitchen, and the Giants won. So now J wants me to get blood transfusions every day. I really need to get him to read Bradford Hill.

June 12, 2013

First contact!

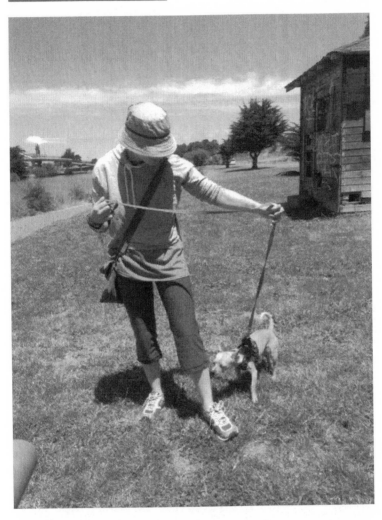

To all you doubters out there, I want you to know that not only am I now a certified dog walker at the animal shelter BUT I achieved this status after only one mentoring session AND my skills with the leash enabled me to leapfrog past the "easier" dogs and I am permitted to walk both "green" and "yellow" dogs! The shelter codes the dogs based on their aggressiveness etc. and most volunteers start out only able to walk the "green" dogs but I am incredibly impressive and amazing and have dog walking skills never before seen at the shelter, or so my mentor clearly seemed to be suggesting when he said "I think you'd be ok with the 'yellow' dogs."

Next stop, orange! It's good to have goals.

In other news, it turns out that having a good amount of blood in your body is very helpful! I have been feeling pretty good post-transfusion. Although this morning I exhausted myself straightening the pillows on the couch so I wonder if I have dropped back down a bit. I've got a MUGA scan tomorrow to make sure my heart is tolerating the poison ok (last scan was normal), and then chemo next week. This will be my 6th and "final" cycle!!! While I don't look forward to the presumably worse cumulative side effects, it will be much easier knowing that this is the last round...at least until someone suggests I do more chemo. I'll have one more PET scan in a few weeks as a final opportunity for chemo to impress us with her accomplishments.

The other exciting development is that we've decided to go to Dana Farber for a multidisciplinary consult. I remain unconvinced that the Kaiser folks will all get together and talk about my case and recommend a specific plan – perhaps my skepticism has something to do with the fact that this hasn't happened. Also, oncologist #2 commented that tumor

95

board was stupid making me think that asking Kaiser folks to get together and talk about me is like asking a bear not to shit in the woods. My oncologist suggested stopping chemo after 4 cycles and then waiting 2 months and rescanning and deciding at that point if surgery and/or XRT makes sense. I'm no oncologist but that doesn't make a lot of sense to me since I was tolerating the chemo ok, and it seemed to be doing something, and if I was going to do that why did I do chemo in the first place? Obviously we haven't gone with that suggestion because we opted to finish the treatment and go through the 6th cycle. Waiting a few months and rescanning may make sense, but I'd like input from DF before potentially losing all the ground gained from doing chemo in the first place. So, I'm all set to see the medical oncologist we've been working with as well as thoracic surgery, general surgery, ortho, and radiation oncology. I'm looking forward to having some cohesive input on next steps. Also, I'm hoping to finally find the apparently elusive cancer center waiting room cucumber water.

June 18, 2013

Close...

Last round of chemo started today, go back tomorrow for the rest of the meds. Hopefully I will just have a somewhat crappy week and then start to come out of it. It's just as well as I have run out of things to eat that I wouldn't mind never eating again (went with Cream of Wheat tonight, excellent choice). That and just in general it's not a super fun experience. Much easier psychologically knowing that this is the last one, at least for now. Once this cycle ends and my counts start to come back up we head to Dana Farber early July for a smorgasbord of appointments. While we are of course looking forward to the end of chemo, it was somewhat easier having a plan and going with it, and now we have to come up with a new one which will likely be a challenge.

Also, J doesn't want my hair to grow back - he likes it that it no longer gets up his nose. While I'm open to discussion, I think he's going to have to deal with that. It's no longer just an aesthetic issue - I can't handle being capable of frying an egg on my scalp.

June 25, 2013

Bone Marrow Appreciation Day

A few weeks ago we learned to appreciate red blood cells and their ability to carry oxygen to tissues. Now that I'm neutropenic, I'm learning to appreciate my white blood cells and their ability to keep me from turning into a mushroom. I realize I've been neutropenic before, but I never knew it and somehow knowing it makes it seem much worse! I felt crappy all weekend and yesterday morning so went in to have my labs checked and since every other time in my life I've seen a WBC of 0.8 and an ANC of 350 it has been associated with a very sick person it was hard to not think that I was about to become one of them. But after the perspective gained from spending the night in a plastic bubble fashioned from the plastic bags one used to get from Target before they started charging for them in Alameda County, I think I may have been overly concerned. So today it's back to playing with cat feces and smearing raw pork on my open wounds.

As an aside, we've determined that people appear intimidated when we tell them that we're going to Dana Farber for a 2nd opinion, so from now on we are going to say that we're going to a cancer center in Boston for a 2nd opinion.

July 9, 2013

Preliminary input

So far doctors from a cancer center in Boston are suggesting "aggressive surveillance" (considered better sounding than "watch and wait") - don't yet know exactly what that means, and more docs to weigh-in, but general idea is scan every few months and if tons of shit shows up, consider chemo again, if nothing happens in 6 months, consider surgery to remove the lesions. The argument is that it's not worth doing surgery now if there's a chance that off chemo the cancer is about to go apeshit because a)surgery won't get everything out and b)it's not great to have just done surgery and then find out that you need to chemo. I guess I'm surprised since I expected they would recommend doing something post-chemo, but it makes sense to me. I don't think this is necessarily good or bad news. More deets to follow after more appointments.

PS it is hot as shit here

July 30, 2013

Now what?

J keeps threatening to eat "several bunches of bananas" which I thought was his solution to stomach upset caused by eating at Taco Bell - which I think counts as a bit more than a passive death wish - but then I realized that the bananas, and not Taco Bell, have been part of his "suicidal ideation with a plan" ever since he heard me say something about potassium and suicide (n.b. that conversation wasn't so much directly cancer-related but came up in discussion about all the terrible things that could happen if I got pregnant - we decided that a stillbirth was the worst possible option and a friend offered to be present in the delivery room and to bring along some potassium chloride).

Now will you stop being bummed that I haven't written lately?

To follow-up on a few loose ends:

1. Cancer center in Boston did NOT have cucumber water but check out the refreshment station!

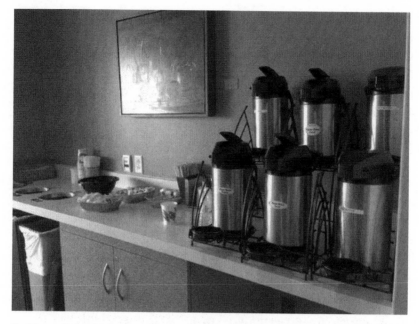

2. I've picked up the dog walking again, though am feeling a bit rusty.

3. My eyelashes are growing back! Their growth skills impress me far more than those of the hair on my head and/or eyebrows. J examines each day but there's not much progress.

As we anticipated, it seems much harder now that chemo is over. And that's not just because I miss all the good things about chemo (I tried to make a list but could never think of anything other than not having to shave and root beer floats being appropriate for each and every meal of the day). And while I'm still waiting on the final word from a cancer center in Boston, it seems likely that the recommendation is to "watch and wait" and rescan in a few months. This means back to work in a few weeks and resume a "normal" life. I'm not saying that J and I are just waiting for me to die, but I will say that sometimes it feels as if we are just waiting for me to get sick, and it doesn't actually help that much to think that we could have the "pleasure" of doing this for 10+ years. I actually looked for advice by googling "dealing with terminal illness" (even though I'm not technically terminal since I don't think I'm going to die in a few weeks or months) - but I couldn't figure out how to exclude the inspirational ones from my search. Jesus, some people sure do try to make the most out of a bad situation. I just feel as if my life circumstances have finally caught up with my disposition.

Apologies for not getting back to all of you amazing, kind, and thoughtful people who have been checking in with us in recent weeks. As this post may suggest, we've been in deep cocoon and not playing well with others these days. In the end, it may turn out to only have to do with how badly the Giants are sucking.

August 10, 2013

We got a dog!

Today we made a rather impulsive decision and adopted Cleo from the animal shelter. The extent of the deliberations were something like:

J: Should we take her home?

Me: Sure.

Since J has not yet gone into anaphylactic shock we feel that we are off to an excellent start! I am somewhat concerned that J will forget all about me now that he has something even smaller and softer around. At least I clean up my own shit, for the most part.

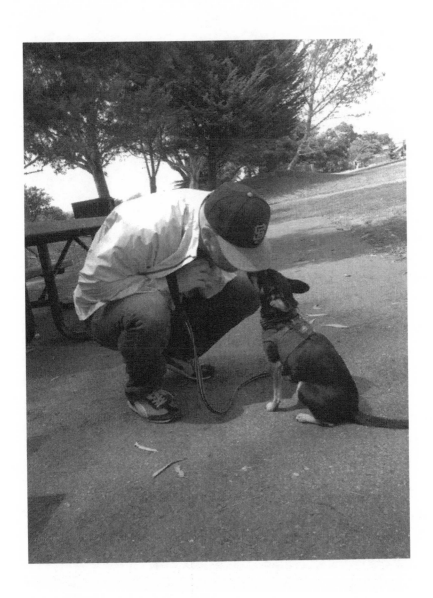

August 13, 2013

Hiatusish?

Now that we are in "aggressive surveillance" mode, I probably won't have many medical updates until my next scan later in the fall so the posts will probably continue on this fairly intermittent schedule.

I do have a medical update about the anterior uveitis (iritis) that a)nobody, even the opthamologists, really cares about because its significance pales in comparison to that of the metastatic cancer and b)deserves the credit for being the reason I found out about the cancer in the first place. I couldn't get off the steroid drops until my 2nd or 3rd round of chemo (which was expected to knock out the inflammation), and then 3 weeks after my last round of chemo it flared again. I managed to get off the drops after a few weeks so I've now had about a week symptom and steroid free, for the first time since December. Apparently it is somewhat unusual to have this sort of nearly chronic iritis. The Kaiser uveitis expert actually volunteered (!) to refer me to the UCSF optho oncologist, which probably has something to do with the fact that she recently finished her fellowship there. I went yesterday and there isn't much new to report - yes it's odd to have this chronic picture, but it's still not likely related to the cancer, and regardless, as long as there is no active inflammation, or the inflammation is controlled with steroid drops, there isn't any reason to try to figure out more about it. If the symptoms recur and steroids don't work, they might consider another tap to see if they find some malignant cells. They don't think it's likely to be paraneoplastic since it's unilateral, and there's no reason to think that there is tumor mass since I don't have other symptoms (proptosis, etc.). In short, nothing new, but still nice to have their input.

Speaking of input from UCSF, next week we are going to UCSF to meet with their sarcoma oncologist. We aren't going for another opinion, we are really just going to meet him to help us decide if we want to transfer our care in 2014. I believe that I can switch my health insurance back to blue shield and then access UCSF. In many ways, I would actually prefer to stay with Kaiser (!) as it is really convenient and efficient (compared to the alternatives) and it will be a pain in the ass to go to UCSF. But if I stay with Kaiser, I'm going to keep wanting input from the cancer center in Boston which could get fairly awkward if/when the oncologist there suggests something with which my Kaiser oncologist does not agree. In anticipation of that inevitability, it might make more sense to switch to UCSF so that the person making the recommendations will be the same person who is implementing them.

In far more important news, Cleo has been an amazingly wonderful addition to our little household! The only bummer is that overnight we now understand how people become crazy about their pets. On more than one occasion, I've had to restrain myself from showing someone a photo of Cleo doing something that is "the cutest thing in the entire world!" We're working on a solution to that problem.

August 16, 2013

Cleo

Getting Cleo has been the best decision we've made in a while. J is very excited to train her so that she's not a "shit stain." He may be getting a bit too much into it since on more than one occasion he has told me that I'm a "good girl" when I've done something he likes. If I can get him to add an edible treat to the verbal reward it wouldn't seem so bad. My only complaint about her is that since she's a girl, it's hard to tell if she's about to pee or take a shit.

For the first time ever, J and I have a facebook account! Well, it's really Cleo's account. Cleo has a very strict friend policy - she only wants friends who want to look at photos of her. https://www.facebook.com/cleo.roikoe

August 20, 2013

Back to the mothership

Went to UCSF yesterday, and despite the oncologist being TWO HOURS (!) late for our appt, we were smitten and I am going to switch care for 2014, assuming the insurance works out. After speaking with him, it seemed clear that we'd be better served at UCSF than at Kaiser. It's not even so much an issue of the quality of the care, but the absence of a collaborative, team approach at Kaiser is what most bothers me. We realize that we'll always have to wait to see him, but it's clearly the cost that we'll have to pay for him to spend as much time with us as we need once it's our turn, and that's well worth the price.

Oh, and he also had 2 Giants pins on his white coat.

I've developed some intermittent neuropathy mostly in my hands/fingers which my Kaiser oncologist said was not likely due to the vincristine since it's so long after the last dose - but UCSF onc. said it most certainly is due to the vincristine damaging my nerves and lowering the threshold for some compressive neuropathy. He also has an interesting theory about the iritis and suggests that it may be due to some sort of auto-immune dysfunction and that the absence of a fully functional immune system may have helped the mesenchymal cs develop. I admit that coming out of anyone else's mouth that would sound insane to me, but when he says it I can believe it's a possibility. He thinks that's more likely than the cancer contributing to the iritis since chondrosarcs are so "bland" and rarely have paraneoplastic manifestations. I'm just happy for a possible explanation that ties the two of them together since it really dulls my Occam's razor to think they are unrelated. He also raised the issue about perhaps taking preventive measures regarding my bone lesions. My chemo-induced menopause adds to the risk of a pathological fracture and there are few things that would fuck me up more right now than breaking my femur (more confirmation that my running days are over). So he is going to speak to the radiation oncologists to see if we should do something now. And I will go back and see him on October after my next scan.

In the meantime, Cleo continues to entertain us - although I'm starting to wonder if she is the one who is training us.

August 21, 2013

Fuck yeah!

On the list of post-cancer diagnosis cliches, doing all those things you've always wanted to do but have never done must be at the top. I've made a few changes - I now throw out socks with holes in them, I no longer clean out moldy mayonnaise jars so that they can be recycled, we have a dog, etc. But today I finally got my first tattoo! It was an idea I toyed with for years but it wasn't until J and I got married that getting one seemed like more than just a thing to do. Tattoos are a big part of his life experience, and I wanted to share that with him. I had a general idea of what I wanted but never felt any urgency to work out the details. As soon as I was diagnosed I really wanted to figure it out. Of course, then I went through chemo and if I learned nothing else from my many years of medical training, I did come out of it all with the idea that it's useful to have a functioning immune system when having needles stuck into your skin. I always wanted a wave, to reflect my love of being in the ocean, but it turns out that all those surfers like being in the ocean too and I didn't want one of their Japanese-style wave tattoos. It was only after I described what I wanted to the tattoo artist that I realized that I was borrowing elements from my engagement ring that J had made and from one of J's tattoos.

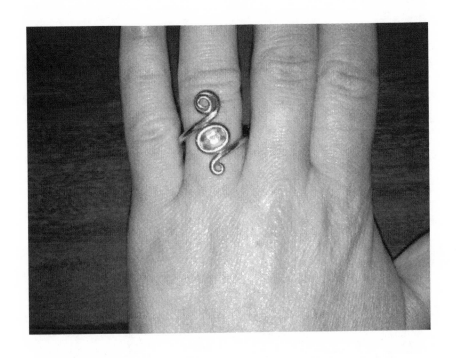

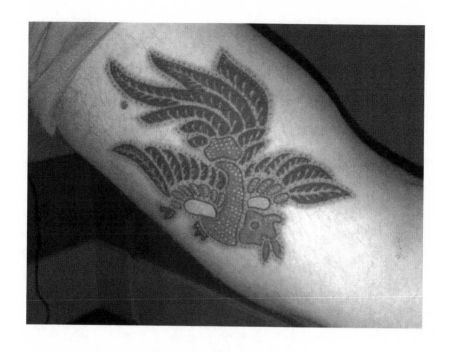

Anyway, here it is, and I love it!

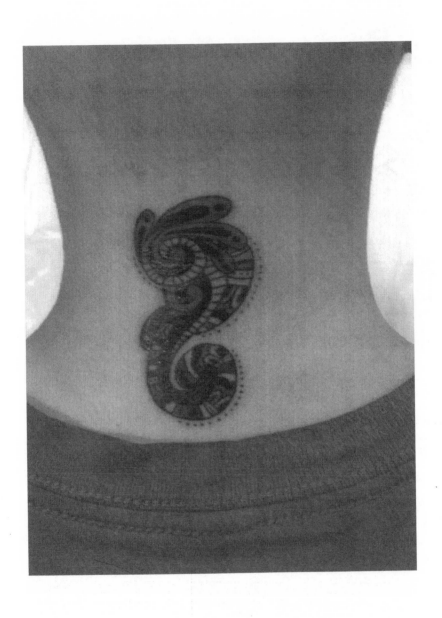

August 30, 2013

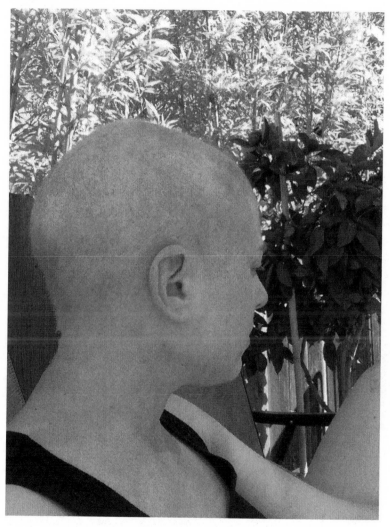

Time for a haircut!

September 2, 2013

Ingredients

for a post-first-day-back-after-6-months-off-work fête:

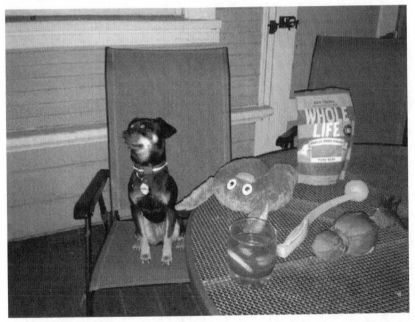

1. Backyard

2. Dog reasonably interested in playing fetch

3. Variety of fetch-oriented toys, including a nasty blue one named 'dodger' designed to be chewed up and spit out, most likely starting in April 2014

4. Dog treats

5. Cocktail (recipe: rye from CBS, boozy cherries from MI, bitters, splash of seltzer from RCC, meyer lemon from backyard, ice-filled freezer, cocktail glass, and appreciation of brown liquor from J)

Many might think that number 6 should be J himself, but J is currently out of town. Those same many might think that J being out of town is a terrible coincidence and that a good marriage would mean that we are both here to deal with this transition together. I maintain that a good marriage is knowing that since my stress about going back to work = J upset because he's stressed that I'm stressed => RJ fight; this is a good time for J to do some favors for others that involve driving 2 cars a total of 4600 miles, so he's doing that.

Two compliments on the shape of my head today! None from patients.

September 5, 2013

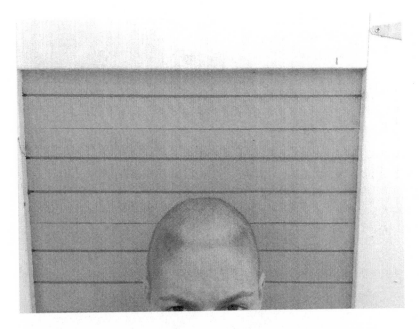

First J was calling me "Friar Tuck" because of my frair-pattern hair growth. And then he changed it to "Friar Wilson" in honor of the tennis ball component to my hair growth in general.

It's a good thing I have a sense of humor.

It's also nice to have eyebrows!

September 13, 2013

Yes, shame is still an option

I got my medical records from an oncology center in Boston, and the orthopedic surgeon (or should I say, the PA with whom he works cause there's no way the orthopedic surgeon wrote that part of the note) misdocumented my intra-residency hospitalization for a periorbital MRSA abscess (it was only mid-occupational medicine fellowship that I realized this was a significant work-related illness!) as a periRECTAL abscess. How humiliating!* Especially since there is no mention an underlying illness that would have predisposed me to getting one so it can just be assumed that I'm disgusting. Even worse, the UCSF oncologist copied the PMH from the ortho note (probably because orthopedic surgeons, and the PAs with whom they work, are recognized for taking and documenting such thorough and accurate histories, never mind that ortho services have been known to request ID consults just so that a thorough history and physical gets documented**) so now my UCSF medical record also includes mention of this perirectal abscess! I know anyone can get a perirectal abscess, and I realize that many, if not most, of the people reading this have probably had one at some point in their lives, but it's still humiliating given the lack of an underlying risk factor other than the implied inability to clean myself.

When I had the very first CXR and it seemed that the mass was most likely a tuberculoma, I thought that it was a perfect medical companion piece to my MRSA abscess as part of my whole "diseases of poverty" oeuvre. At least if I had TB, the

117

perirectal abscess would have a poetic component to it, but with (non-GI) cancer it's just sad.

*Apologies to anybody, and everybody, who has ever had a perirectal abscess. I'm just going to assume that you agree with me that even though there is nothing actually shameful about having one, it's still embarrassing. I think that's just how most of us would feel if we had one.

**Apologies to all orthopedic surgeons, and the PAs with whom they work, for the generalizations. But I am upset about this unnecessary shame!

September 21, 2013

A funny thing happened...animal shelter

When we adopted Cleo, there was another dog we were considering adopting, Frankie, a 3 year-old stray, lab/pit bull mix (in other words, the dog version of J). I was somewhat partial to him, I must admit, as he was a bit bigger and more my "style" (historically). But Cleo was a better choice for a lot of reasons and Frankie was somewhat dog-reactive which was concerning. He was also really sweet so it seemed like just a matter of time before he was adopted. Fast-forward to this week and Frankie is still at the shelter and about to be put down. So, uhm,

118

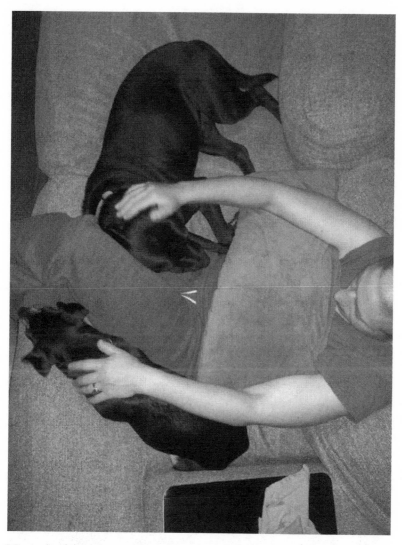

Now, in fairness to our sanity, we didn't outright adopt him, we are fostering. If all goes well we hope to keep him, but we thought that as wacky as it was to get a 2nd dog right now, it seemed even wackier to do an outright adoption. So far he and Cleo are getting along pretty well. We will be taking him to BADRAP (http://www.badrap.org/) classes - they make their classes available to put bull breeds when they are in the shelter and they continue to be available if you adopt from the shelter - pretty cool.

Here are some better photos of him. I think he'll have to wait to make sure he's a permanent addition to the household before he gets his own facebook page. But for now, interested parties can follow his exploits on Cleo's page (https://www.facebook.com/cleo.roikoe).

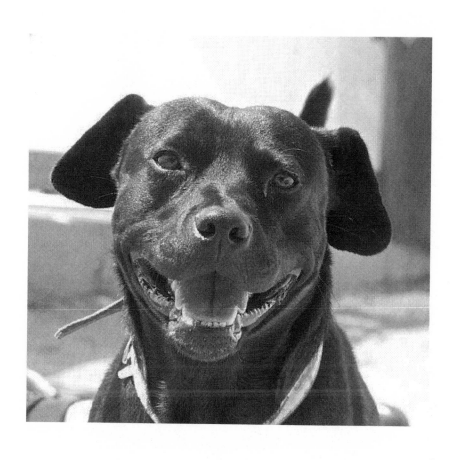

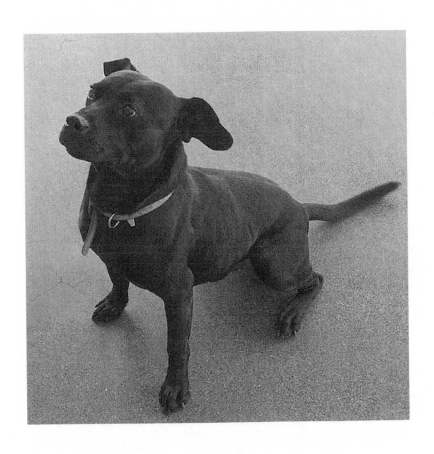

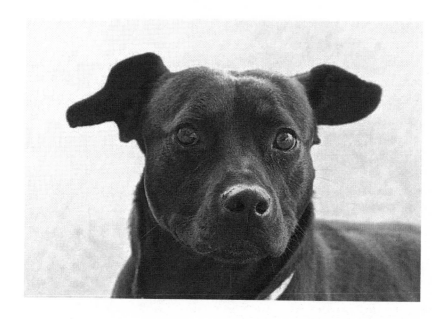

October 2, 2013

Amazeballs!

PET scan today showed no change from 3 months ago! No new lesions, no change in size, even the metabolic activity is still reduced from pre-chemo levels! As J said, this is the second best news we've had all day (he got out of a speeding ticket this morning). We meet with the oncologists next week but presumably the plan will be to chillax and repeat the scan in 3 months.

Hmm, maybe I should stop eating cupcakes every day.

In other news, we adopted Frankie on Monday so we've gone from zero to two dogs in 6 weeks. On the one hand, I couldn't find anything that said it was a good idea to bring two dogs into the home without more time for the first dog to get adjusted, on the other hand, metastatic mesenchymal chondrosarcoma. Things are going well so far. But let's just say that nighttime crate training efforts have been thwarted by J's discovery that dogs are warm and soft combined with what have apparently been allergy shots containing magic beads (2013 has really been "The Year of Living Big Pharma"). He bought Cleo a peacoat yesterday, with a hood, sadly (fortunately?) it didn't fit. I guess 2013 could also be "The Year of Becoming Crazy Dog People." We still bathe, but I can see how that may start to become tedious at some point.

The photo from the last post is so mediocre that I feel compelled to provide a better one. And yes, Frankie's tail is in between Cleo's legs!

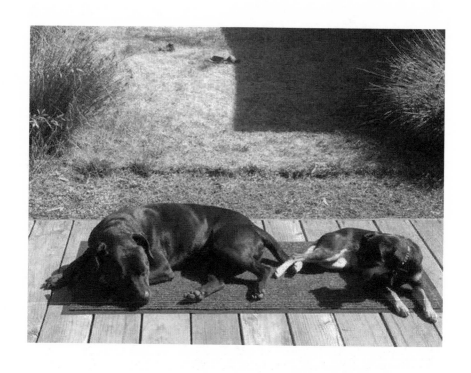

November 13, 2013

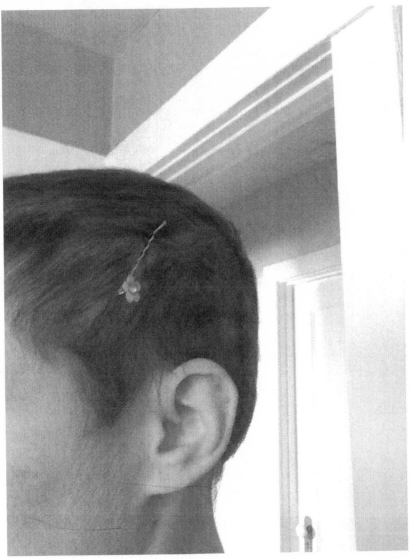

File under…

Meaning well but just not knowing what to say.

A woman at work welcomed me back and said that having cancer must give me perspective on what's important in life. She then said she wished she could have that sort of perspective. I told her I hoped she could get it without having cancer.

Good thing I still have these bobby pins (from 2nd grade?!?!?) - it is a challenge to keep the hair out of my eyes. Just half an inch away from being super on-trend rather than super cancery.

Still in that "but for the chest xray I wouldn't know about this" phase - which is great. Sure, cancer bone pain is a great way to keep my narcs supply steady, but I still prefer being asymptomatic. Scan again early 2014 and go from there. We are in the midst of J's "bday month" (which somehow spans 6 weeks) so I'm pretty busy "celebrating" that and worrying that I haven't bought him enough presents (he likes his presents the way he likes the amount of time he is to be celebrated - excessive).

Fortunately it's kind of cute. Plus, he told me that up to 1/3rd of his presents can be for the dogs.

January 10, 2014

My body is a wonderland!

Well, except for all the miscarriages and the rare cancer.

But other than that, this protoplasm is friggin amazing. Had my 3 month PET scan this week and things are pretty stable - no new lesions and nothing is larger. If this keeps up I may have to become less self-absorbed. Obviously the detox massage I had a few weeks ago worked. Or perhaps it was my neighbor's suggestion that I check out hemp oil ("that stuff is amazing, it cures every kind of cancer!") that made the difference (although since I didn't actually "check out hemp oil" I fear there is a flaw in that logic, somewhere, deep down, there just must be a tiny little flaw). But how nice to find out that the world is actually very simple!

The lesions are more metabolically active than they were 3 months ago but it's not clear if that's clinically meaningful or just due to the fact that this scan was not done with a TI-99/4A.

Ha!

I don't mean to be an academic medicine snob but when you look at the images from this scan and the ones from the scan done at Kaiser it's like the difference between the special effects in Clash of the Titans and the special effects from a movie with much less shitty special effects.

There is also a little spot in my frontal lobe that my oncologist is so sure is nothing that he doesn't even recommend an MRI but it is exciting to think about the possibility of brain mets. I'm no oncologist but clearly having tumor cells in your brain has got to be super awesome And if I do end up with some frontal lobe disinhibition I think we can all agree that it will just make me more fun. I sure won't need anyone doing jazz hands on my behalf! But the oncologist isn't that worried about it so I'm not going to give it a second thought.

Oh, wait, too late!

Not clear what the next steps are - plan to get input from an oncologist in Boston (my SF oncologist's suggestion - what a concept!), likely will talk to radiation oncology and surgeons about whether a combo of interventions makes sense. I assume/hope this will all get figured out in the next few weeks.

Speaking of SF oncology, nice digs! Not the oncology office at Mt Zion which has a cattle holding pen feel to it, but the new radiology dept at Mission Bay. The best part is they give you a gown, pants, a robe, AND socks! All that plus the blanket straight out of the warmer and all I was missing was a nice mug of hot cocoa - I cannot imagine being more comfortable while awaiting news about the havoc cancer cells are wreaking on my body! Here's my attempt to capture the cozy bounty.

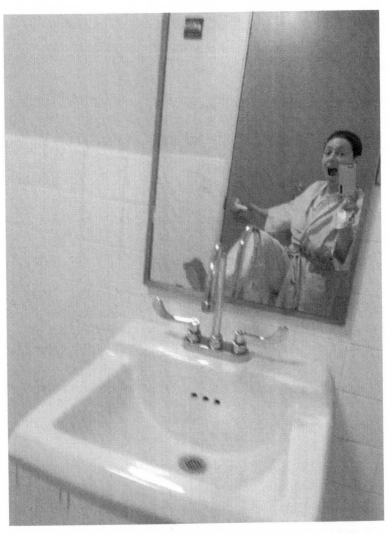

But I do worry about what will happen if I end up coding at 5:30, or on the weekend.

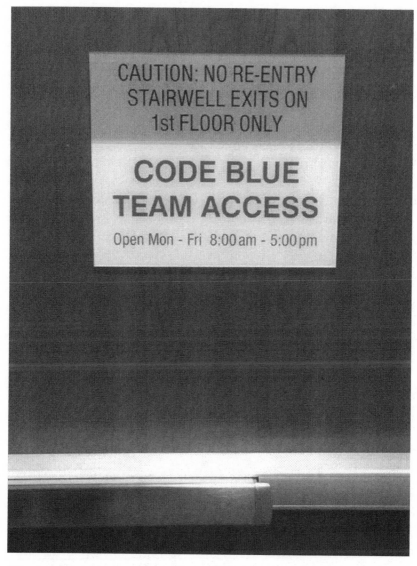

"Such a shame, she was such a nice girl, if only she had timed things differently."

February 26, 2014

Clear as mud

It's officially official that nobody is willing or able to make sense of the increased metabolic activity seen on my Jan. PET scan (compared to the Oct. scan done on a different machine). I don't blame them - what would we do with the info anyway? Nobody is going to discount it entirely and suggest we start carving away at all my mets, and nobody is going to say it is so clearly problematic that we should start chemo again. So we wait until the next scan in April and go from there.

I spoke with both my UCSF oncologist and DFG (I'm going back to "Dana Farber Guy" since "A cancer center in Boston was getting a bit cumbersome". I do need a catchy nickname for the UCSF guy - I am accepting suggestions.) I spoke to them both on the same day and it is interesting, though not surprising, that their opinions about next steps differ slightly. I didn't bother pitting one opinion against the other; there's no reason to try to get them to resolve their differences at this point since there is no decision that actually needs to be made.

DFG: He is a bit more conservative. If the next scan shows a bunch of new mets, or existing mets are larger, then chemo. If there is one more met, or some other signs of increased activity (not metabolic activity but new lesions or growth) that aren't widespread, then talk about chemo. No new lesions, no increase in size of existing lesions, metabolic activity be dammed, then wait 6 months for the next scan. His general take on surgery and radiation is that they might be useful in the setting of my having symptoms without evidence of more widespread disease. I'm not sure when/if that scenario might ever occur but I get his point since there is no evidence that taking everything out is going to improve my survival and it's certainly not going to improve my quality of life at this point since there are few symptoms that need to be improved upon (left hip pain but I rarely even take an NSAID for that).

UCSF guy: He agrees that new mets = chemo though I get the impression that he would suggest chemo for even one new met whereas DFG is not so clear on that. If things are stable in April then scan again in late summer which will be a year post-chemo. If things are stable then consider surgery/radiation to take everything out for "cure," Yes, he uses the word "cure." He is the only person to use that word so I'm not exactly doing the layout for the "I had surgery and all I got was this lousy cure" tshirt, but I figure the people who read this blog who are interested in my well-being will like to hear that word. Those who read the blog just to know what's up in hip metastatic cancer blogging may not care so much.

Everyone agrees that it's good news that nothing really changed in the 6 months after chemo. Unexpectedly, I did not get much of an answer to the question about how I'm supposed to live the rest of my life. DFG again quoted studies in which 30% of patients with mesenchymal chondrosarcoma lived more than 10 years and obviously the hope is that I'm in that category.

In the meantime, the hair is officially styley (next stop, fauxhawk!) and pitchers and catchers reported about 2 weeks ago and we are off to spring training in 10 days!

March 6, 2014

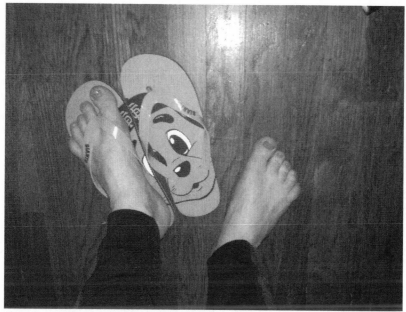

Who's ready for Spring Training?

Yes, those are children's flip flops - but at least I had to get an XL!

Too bad I have hair, now I will never get my Make-A-Wish dream of rescuing Lou Seal from Crazy Quilt and getting to snuggle with him.

We'll always have FurCon.

And yes, the third toe on my left foot is shorter than the 2nd toe. That and my tumors are the basis of my Body Dysmorphic Disorder.

April 8, 2014

This is the kind of shit

that is somehow both not that big a deal and really stressful. Kind of a cancer-play on the old "necessary and sufficient" concept. I'm supposed to have my next PET scan this week and get the results next week, and I just found out that the insurance won't cover it! According to the physician (yes, an MD, not someone without any clinical training!) who reviewed the request for a PET, I *had* chondrosarcoma and the PET is to see if it has come back. Since I've had no recent treatment, or testing, or problems, there is no reason to believe that the cancer has returned.

Hallelujah! I've been cured!

According to Anthem Blue Cross (names have been changed to protect the innocent), the PET is considered investigational because there is no evidence to suggest that the cancer has come back.

For those of you who have not been paying attention, I hate to break the news to you this way, but the cancer and the mets haven't gone anywhere. I've had some reduction in metabolic activity but no change in size. So not only am I not in remission, the changes I've had are not ones that are going to be detected on a (less expensive) scan like a CT scan - the only way of tracking this is by looking at metabolic activity and PET's the way to do that.

136

While it is hardly critical that I get scanned this week (or next week, or even the week after next), I do some prep work around the time of the scan and I don't appreciate a last minute change of schedule. Sure, the work I've done (screw with J's calendar so he's confused about which day it is and when the scan is actually occurring, stock fridge with beer, prepare cocooning supplies such as ice cream, pajamas, clean sheets, and crime dramas, prep dogs for hibernation, organize life so interaction with outside world is unnecessary and thus likelihood of arrest due to "excessive sarcasm" is low, etc.) will "keep" for a few more days (or weeks), but this still stresses me out!

I'm already working on the appeal and I've spoken to my oncologist and assume this will be resolved quickly since most issues with insurance companies are pretty easy to resolve once you point out that the insurance co. is wrong and their decision is illogical. But for some reason my desire for a stiff drink remains high.

April 11, 2014

All clear!

PET scan approved, results next week, stay tuned.

April 16, 2014

Stable!

Lesions are relatively stable (some increased metabolic activity which isn't freaking anyone out) - nothing new. Next step is for UCSF/DFG meeting of the minds to discuss next steps. I hope to know more in a week or so.

Now I can replace my torn autoclavable hospital shoes! I wasn't going to bother if the scan was bad.

May 21, 2014

Tie a pink ribbon

Man, breast cancer is clearly the popular cancer. Check out this intake form for physical therapy - how can it be that the ONLY cancer they care about is breast cancer? Seriously, I promise, my awareness has been raised.

Diagnosis / Medical History

Patient Denies PMH	☐	Coronary Artery Disease	☐	Kidney Stone	☐
Arrhythmia	☐	Diabetes Type I	☐	Migraine	☐
Arthritis	☐	Diabetes Type II	☐	Myocardial Infarction	☐
Asthma	☐	Diverticulitis	☐	Pancreatitis	☐
Autoimmune disease	☐	Ectopic Pregnancy	☐	Peptic Ulcer Disease	☐
Back disorder	☐	Fibromyalgia	☐	Psychiatric Disorder	☐
Bowel obstruction	☐	Gallbladder Disease	☐	Renal Disease	☐
Breast cancer	☐	Gastroesophageal Reflux (GERD)	☐	Respiratory Disease	☐
Cerebral vascular accident (Stroke)	☐	Hepatitis	☐	Seizures	☐
CHF	☐	HIV	☐	Substance Abuse	☐
COPD	☐	Hypertension (High Blood Pressure)	☐	Tuberculosis	☐

Other Problems

Clostridium Difficile	☐
Depression	☐
Ear Infection	☐
MDRO (Multi-Drug Resistant Organism, e.g., MRSA, VRE)	☐
Osteopenia/Osteoporosis	☐
Urinary/Fecal Incontinence	☐

If you have been diagnosed with any of the previous diagnoses or had any of the prob **please describe if the condition is active or if it is resolved.**

Anyhoo, DFG and UCSF guy finally communicated with each other and their recommendation is as I suspected - if it ain't broke, don't fuck with it.

Since:

1) I'm still relatively asymptomatic

and

2) there's no evidence to suggest that intervening (radiation, surgery) will improve my survival

and

3) intervening presumably can't improve my quality of life given the absence of symptoms

139

and

4) intervening has its own host of potential bad consequences

I should just keep on keeping on with this "active surveillance." But instead of another scan in 3 months wait until September (5 months) for the next scan. If my symptoms (intermittent left hip pain) worsen or new symptoms develop I imagine they may be more inclined to intervene.

Until then, I just plan to eat a lot of stone fruit.

Peace Out.

June 18, 2014

Unsuccessful distraction

Started to watch Murder in the First since a)it's a crime drama and b)that's pretty much all I want to watch these days. Also, it seemed fun that it was based in SF. And yes, I knew the premise, so it wasn't a surprise, but I couldn't get past the 12 minute mark when the detective's wife (dying of late stage pancreatic cancer) was set-up in home hospice. Jeez, I never knew I was such a friggin wimp! Fortunately I had the good sense to make sure that J wasn't watching with me. Maybe she will die quickly so I can try the show again.

I guess there is always "Chasing Life" which really seems like it would be a good fit for me. I really like the image of the lemons in the coffin - cancer-flavored lemonade is so delicious.

October 3, 2014

Here we go

Welcome back to the blog - probably. Most recent PET scan, 5 months since the last one, showed no new lesions (yay!) but 3 out of 4 lesions are larger and more metabolically active (left hip lesion is about the same). I have been having fairly constant, usually mild, left hip pain that is worse with activity, weight-bearing, etc. (but since I almost never put weight on my left leg this is a total non-issue) so UCSF oncologist referred me to rad onc to discuss whether xrt is a good idea. I have an appt mid-October. UCSF onc. is also suggesting 3 cycles of chemo (ifosfamide, etoposide) followed by surgery to remove the lung and pancreas lesions, and another 3 cycles of chemo. This would probably add up to about a year of treatment.

Yikes!

I've sent the scans to DFG and want his input too. He has always been more conservative though I guess I am expecting him to come up with a similar plan. As you may or may not recall, this was the plan a while ago - if things are stable, take them out. But I think we kind of forgot this was the plan so it has taken some time to wrap our heads around this new potential reality.

What will make this chemo extra fun is 1)it's in SF 2)it's an inpatient regimen (4-5 days in the hospital the first week of each 4 week cycle) AND 3)I'll get to be on a UCSF medicine service (with oncology consult) - 14L! At least it's not CRI. I plan to spend a lot of time working with the medical students. I can think of nothing I'd rather do in the midst of my chemo than educate the future physicians of America. I have a functional murmur that will make for a fascinating physical exam finding.

I know, it's terrible, I should be much more supportive of medical training than the average person with mesenchymal chondrosarcoma. But, honestly, if I could cash-in my professional courtesy chits I'd skip med students, residents, fellows, etc. I know how the sausage is made…insert clever play on an idiomatic expression or hilarious mixed metaphor here.

J, naturally, is ecstatic. It turns out his calling is taking care of me so he will be in his element. He is already dusting off the blender and the other day I found him ironing my sweatpants. The only problem is that if treatment starts this fall it will likely interfere with his "birthday month."

It will be a few more weeks before any of this is figured out. But for those of you who enjoyed my musings on food that doesn't seem disgusting in the midst of chemo, you may be in for an entertaining 2015.

November 7, 2014

And so it begins!

Again.

First day of XRT (radiation, gotta keep up with the lingo non-med folks) today. It is supposed to be five consecutive days but because of the holiday on Tuesday I start today and finish next Friday - isn't it supposed to be a bit more precise than that???? They tattooed me for the sake of precision, but UCSF's high regard for veterans, which I'm sure is evidenced by all sorts of things, means no xrt on Tuesday.

The radiation oncologist gave new meaning to the term "MD, PhD." We got him to say "I don't know how to respond to that" twice during one appointment. The first time was after he asked if we had kids and we explained our situation (miscarriages, chemo, the god we don't believe in punishing us, etc.) and the second time was when I told him that if we could arrange the simulation appointment (which involves a CT scan) to be on the day of a Giants playoff game (all-day, free parking for the CT scan right across the street from the ballpark!) it would make the whole cancer thing worthwhile. As CF, one of the two best MD, PhDs I know, pointed out, we should have just told him to say whatever his microchip's human program told him to say. Fortunately he's not the one we will ever have to talk to about hospice.

And finally, after 6 weeks, I spoke to my oncologist who spoke to DFG. Part of the issue is that DFG is no longer DFG - he left Dana Farber! He provided some input this time around but I'm assuming he's not going to be in the picture going forward as I think he moved to WA and left academic medicine for family reasons. Apparently he had the same idea as my oncologist (decent nickname still pending) which is that if we want to be aggressive do some xrt (especially since I'm having pain) then 2-3 cycles of inpatient chemo, and if it is "working" (defined as no new lesions, nothing

143

larger, at the very least no progression but realistically probably less metabolic activity and/or smaller are key - not that they've ever gotten smaller with chemo) consider surgery (perhaps going after the lung first since that's "easiest" - that's why we have so many lobes since it's so easy to live without one of them, then go for the pancreas lesion), then another 3 cycles of chemo. The whole plan would take at least a year assuming everything goes well and no complications. And since there is no "guarantee" that this will prolong my life, or improve my quality of life, since there is so little data/so few patients on which to base this course of action, it is of course entirely up to me and if treatment seems super unpleasant it wouldn't be unreasonable to let the cancer take its course. But since I really don't have anything better to do I figure why not? I just need to remind myself that god never gives us more than we can handle.

And whenever god closes a door he opens a window.

And god works in mysterious ways.

And jesus loves me.

Unfortunately for the planner in me, everything is going to happen bit by bit. So I am not scheduled for chemo; I'm just supposed to call my oncologist when I'm done with XRT (in a week). Assuming I tolerate it ok and want to proceed with chemo I will be scheduled for that 1-2 weeks later - probably first week of December.

Speaking of people to whom I wish I could ensure badness befalls, top of my list right now is the super obnoxious flight attendant who was so obnoxious that I approached her at the end of the flight to tell her that her obnoxiousness marred the trip I took in anticipation of a year of radiation, chemo, and surgery for my metastatic bone cancer and that I hoped she enjoyed her power trip. That should have been enough but her response was so insufficient that it prompted me to tell her that she gave all plus-sized waitresses a bad name. Not my typical retort but I was desperate and would have given anything to figure out how to make her cry. Now my only option is to submit an online complaint which I'm sure will be very gratifying.

November 10, 2014

A collection of annoying things

found in the XRT changing room

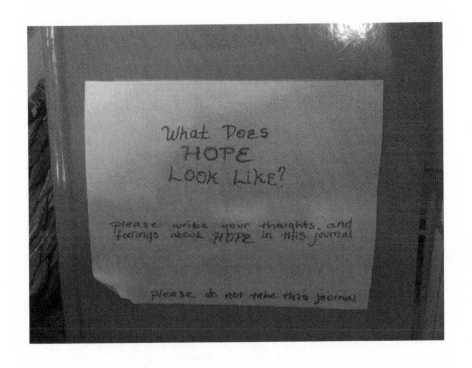

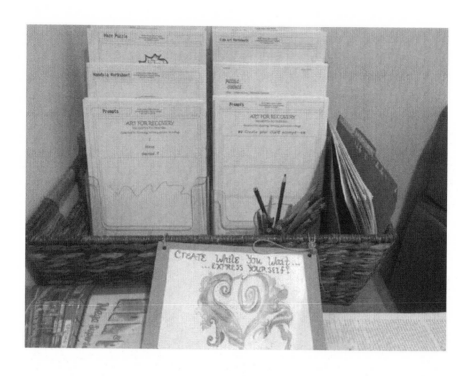

WHAT CANCER CANNOT DO:
CANCER IS SO LIMITED...
IT CANNOT CRIPPLE LOVE.
IT CANNOT SHATTER HOPE.
IT CANNOT DISSOLVE FAITH.
IT CANNOT DESTROY PEACE.
IT CANNOT KILL FRIENDSHIP.
IT CANNOT SUPPRESS MEMORIES.
IT CANNOT SILENCE COURAGE.
IT CANNOT INVADE THE SOUL.
IT CANNOT STEAL ETERNAL LIFE.
IT CANNOT CONQUER THE SPIRIT.

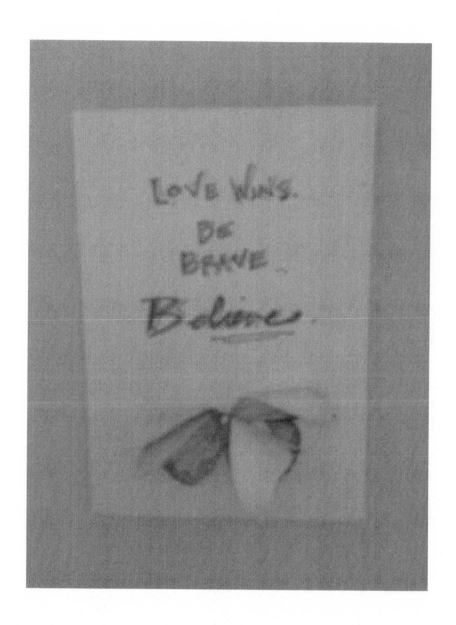

November 22, 2014

The game's afoot

We met with my oncologist yesterday and chemo is on - start the second week of December with 5 nights inpatient. As a bonus he will be on service that week. I warned him that I will likely be extra obnoxious to the med students rather than extra understanding and he seemed fine with that. It would probably be more fun in the spring when I'd be more likely to have an obnoxious, showy, gunner subI to torment. The plan is 2 cycles of chemo (each cycle is a month with 5 nights inpatient) and then a PET scan. If the PET scan shows improvement (nothing new, nothing larger, nothing more metabolically active, and at least some reduction in metabolic activity though size reduction is preferable) then probably surgery (followed by more chemo).

Radiation went fine though it has exacerbated my hip pain - which they warned me was likely to happen before it improves. J seems to be having difficulty with my limping around. He just told me that he isn't going to talk to me if I don't stop limping. We are both curious to see whether his theory that coddling the hip pain will just encourage it is correct. A little reverse psychology seems like as good a strategy as any.

November 23, 2014

Who knew?

Somehow we got nearly 30 minutes into Dallas Buyers Club before it occurred
to either one of us that a movie about AIDS in the 80's was going to be a movie about death. You'd think we were new at this cancer thing. Oh well, on to a crime drama.

December 8, 2014

Hmmm....

What does it mean when you are on your way to chemo and a black cat crosses your path to take a loose shit in your yard?

Can't be good.

December 9, 2014

Musings

27 hours in to my 120hr hospital stay.

Conclusions so far:

1. It is in fact weird to be hospitalized at the same hospital where I used to work, on the same service, and floor, with the

same issues, that I used to have to address as a medicine intern/resident.

2. On a related note, it is odd that my medicine attending was an intern when I was a senior resident, not that either of us remembers the other, or that her presence is especially relevant cause the onc consult runs the show.

3. My counts started low (ABC 3.1 and ANC 1.7!) presumably from the xrt, but onc isn't that worried about it and it doesn't hold up the chemo or anything.

4. I got "lucky" and ended up with a palliative care room which has more space, and furniture, and extra big windows. We were able to reassure ourselves that it was random and not a reflection of how they feel about my prognosis.

5. I'm recording my own I's and O's - well, really just the O's! I am trying to do a really good job!

6. 1mg of lorazepam still knocks me out for several hours - good - so I haven't yet developed tolerance. J claims that I fell asleep while hugging him goodbye but I have no proof of that!

7. Tomorrow I'm hoping J can sweet-talk an RN into letting Cleo visit. I realize it's a long shot. Frankie would do great with the people but the slippery floors would freak him out. They have a therapy dog over in the children's hospital, why not here???

Hopefully this will get more entertaining as the week progresses, but I was warned that it's a pretty boring hospital stay.

December 10, 2014

It was bound to happen eventually

Like many honest physicians before me, I finally gave in to the lure of Big Pharma. The volunteers came around with Genentech sponsored blankets, and one was SF Giants, and I said yes, and now it is around my shoulders!!! This is the first pharma gift I've accepted! What's next? Year supply of pens? Dinner at a snazzy restaurant? A trip to Hawaii? Will my ethical commitments ever return or are they just another in the long list of cancer-related casualties?

But look how nice it is, here, modeled by my IV pole! And it was handmade my someone at Genentech and doesn't say Genentech on it so that seems so much better.

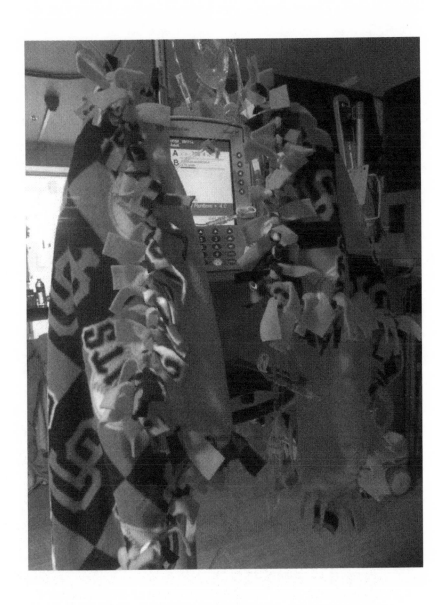

Did I mention that it has fringe? And it is double-layered!

Nothing much to report, I haven't been feeling too poorly and have not tried to claw my face off due to boredom. I am doing an exemplary job recording my urinary output and have no doubt that if awards were given for precision and accuracy I would be in the top 10, at UCSF, for 2014. My dependance on lorazepam seems to be a ways off as the 1mg I took yesterday apparently resulted in my having a number of conversations that I completely forgot about until I was reminded of them today. And in dog news, I passed by a room with a small, white, fluffy dog on the bed so I'm thinking this could happen! And J and I tested out the (surprisingly comfortable) hospital bed which is downright snugglecious so I'm thinking a sleepover is a possibility!

Assuming this "storm of a decade" doesn't get in the way...

December 11, 2014

Inpatient Haiku

BF4ever!
IV pole, bound to
You and your power craving.
But you light the loo!

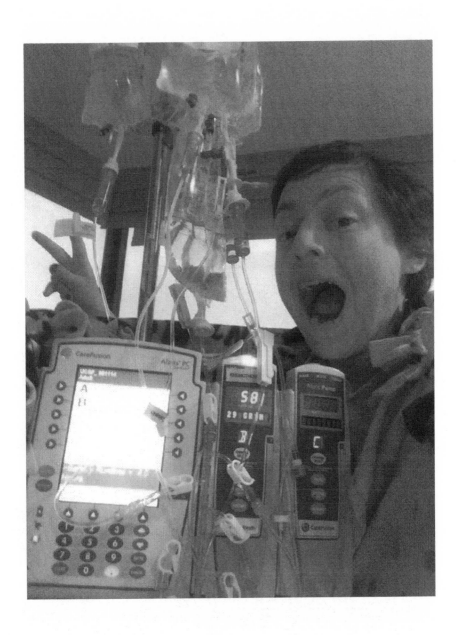

Perhaps I am going a bit stir crazy. Three nights down, 3 days and 2 nights to go.

December 16, 2014

Don't believe the hype!

6 days/5 nights in the hospital is worse than 2 days as an outpatient! I'm not sure why I believed them when they said this regimen is tolerated better than the one I did last year. Maybe the meds themselves are tolerated better - but they are still only given for 2 days whereas I got these meds over 5 days. And the hospital is a bit rough. Although maybe the issue is that this is now my 7th round of chemo rather than my 1st, and I just had XRT, so I'm going into this a bit beat up. In fact, I was a tad neutropenic when chemo started. And yes, everybody in the hospital was fantastic, and I got used to the superfluous medicine team and even tolerated not one, but two, presentations by pharmacy students about the service they provide where they put together a list of all the meds you're supposed to take and when and why and laminate it and call you on the phone and…it really is a fantastic service I just don't think that I need it!
I continue to stay true to my size and be completely floored by what are supposed to be adult-sized doses of meds. I got some prochlorperazine at 9pm and was essentially unconscious until 3pm the next day. Unconscious except for getting up to urinate a liter every 90 minutes. At first I thought my kidneys were going balls to the wall before crashing, but as it turns out, my expert urine output

recordings were to blame! Well, not my
expert UO recordings *per se* but the lack of matched expertise
in recording my In's so it looked like I was putting out 8L to
every 4L was taking in.

I've been home since Saturday night and mostly have been
making up for missed meals and trying to keep up with the
small amount of exercise they recommend (3 x 10 minute
walks a day). I've had to sub a few things for the walks. For
instance, I was craving pancakes and made the batter, but
then was too tired to finish cooking them and J had to take
over. So I decided that counted as a 10 minute walk. And
yesterday, when we spent an absurd 3 hours going to SF to
get an injection that Frankie (the less sharp of our 2 dogs)
could have been trained to give me with about 4 pieces of
dehydrated lamb lung and 5 minutes, merely because of a
classic discharge planning mishap - I decided that counted as
a 10 minute walk. I did also count eating two helpings of
Chinese food for dinner last night as a 10 minute walk and
perhaps that's stretching it - but I went into the kitchen and
fixed the 2nd plate for myself!

The only symptom I really mind is the nausea. The fatigue is
pretty profound (let's just say it's a good thing that pancake
batter isn't supposed to be well mixed), but at least it doesn't
involve nausea and vomiting. Although this round I've
started to wonder if there is a fuzzy border between fatigue
and nausea and I'm not happy about that discovery at all. The
shot I got yesterday is pegfilgrastim so my neutrophil count
should be coming up and the fatigue should get better. J likes
to ask about all the
neutrophils and netrobobs and neutromikes and neutradaves a
nd how many of them there are.

158

At this point, J and I are just so deliriously happy that I'm home, and feeling reasonably ok, that we are oddly in much better shape then we've been in for most of the past year. Looking back on the time in between chemo, it was moderately crappy. I guess we should have been loving life but mostly we were just waiting for the next scan to show progression, or, best case scenario, not much progression so that we could start treatment again. I found myself nearly missing the "fun" we had during chemo when we hung out, did what we were up for doing, and ate as deliciously as I could tolerate. Now we can try to get back to that time where it's pretty clear what we're supposed to be doing.

Vive la chemotherapy!

Well, not really, just in case anyone in a position of power is reading this…

January 5, 2015

Round 2

Back in the hospital for the 2nd cycle; same plan as last time with 5 nights inpatient so should be out on Saturday...not that I'm counting the days or anything.

January 10, 2015

Lessons Learned

6 days is a really long time in the hospital.

Yes, I realize that 7 days is longer, as is 8, but 6 is still pretty darn long.

Also, when you are getting chemo and you start to feel a little nauseated you should take the extra anti-emetics rather than see if it will pass - it's not as if the car you are riding in is about to stop. I did much better on this issue this time.

That's all I've learned from this hospital stay. Overall it has been a shockingly unproductive 6 days with little to show for myself. Last chemo is starting now and I should go home late tomorrow so there isn't much time left to really make something of my time here.

The third cycle is tentatively scheduled for a month from now but I'll have another PET scan before then to make sure this is working. At times it is hard to remember that I am rooting for it to work so that I can do this another 4 times.

January 10, 2015

Fun & Games

Carefully measuring urine output in a dark bathroom in the middle of the night while tethered to an IV pole and slightly snowed on benzos is all fun and games until you get urine on your pajamas.

January 10, 2015

Freedom!

I offered to drink the last 100mL but they wouldn't go for it.

January 30, 2015

Yay!

Turns out the chemo is doing something! PET scan this week showed "marked" reduction in metabolic activity especially in the bone lesions and we met with my oncologist today who was very pleased, and surprised, by the response. We celebrated by taking a 2 ½ hour nap on the couch with the dogs since neither one of us slept well last night. Then I woke up and drank a lot of root beer since "dental health" is low on my list of priorities. We really know how to live it up over here.

Nobody cares much about the size of the lesions at this point but lung one is slightly smaller and pancreas one is slightly larger but that may be due to necrosis. Now the plan is for 2 more cycles and then rescan. This should make it a bit easier to go back to the hospital on Monday but it still sucks a fair bit! I am never doing non-baseball season chemo again - not unless I can get Jon Miller to come sit next to me in the hospital and provide play-by-play.

February 5, 2015

Third verse

Same as the first...

More chemo, more reasonably controlled nausea, more urinating 8 liters/day, more somehow managing to spend 6 days in the hospital not doing anything with mental faculties mostly intact, nothing new to report. The relatively impressively diverse menu has started to get a bit stale this time around. Fortunately J came through with a long trek for some delicious matzah ball soup to change things up. Back on a teaching service this time, blech, but they are mostly

162

leaving me alone. It is weird that I've passed 3 attendings I know from residency (including the one who helpfully suggested I make my presentations more "dynamic" which prompted my co-intern to offer to do jazz hands while I spoke) while doing my laps in the hallway. I haven't bothered to say hello since they wouldn't remember me even if I were not disguised as a cancer patient.

48 hours to go, then one more cycle, then...

February 6, 2015

Hrmph.

I may have been grumpy today, and told J not to bother visiting me, but then he came anyway, apparently because he is immune to my first-grade antics, and then I was less grumpy after he came.

Hrmph.

February 7, 2015

Going home!

In 7 hours...still have to get some meds and a blood transfusion. My hemoglobin isn't quite at their transfusion threshold (7) but it's gonna be in a few days and it's kind of a pain in the ass to get back here for a transfusion. Besides, last time I got a transfusion it made me feel so much better I was considering setting up a private medical practice where I just transfuse people, and give them steroid and B12 injections.

Exciting news in the world of my urine output - I've stopped measuring! For the past 48 hours I've just been estimating. For one thing, the "hat" is annoying, and for another, nobody really gives a shit. They just want to make sure that I am generally putting out about as much as I take in. And the answer is, yes, but only after I puff up for the first 3 days. This has dramatically improved my quality of life in the hospital. I would say it has improved it at least 20%.

I may have been overly obnoxious to the med student - yesterday he asked me to tandem walk - even worse, he asked me to tandem walk when he wasn't there and to "report back" to him. I'm not sure why that seems worse but it really does. Maybe because it partially acknowledges the absurdity of his asking me to tandem walk which makes it that much worse than if he believed it was a reasonable request. I refused. It's not his fault, I know, and if I ever saw his resident or attending (1 visit in 6 days) I would love to give them both a feedback sandwich. "On the one hand, I'm sure you are a really good resident/attending. On the other hand, it is fucking idiotic that you assigned a med student to me both because I'm a shitty case for a med student and because it reflects a lack of professional curtesy that you make my stay here more annoying than it needs to be. But overall I'm sure you are a really good resident/attending." They're all really careful to call me "doctor," which I don't give a shit about. The professional curtesy I would like is to have a little bit of the bullshit stripped away and daily visits from a med student who is going to listen to my lungs and ask me to tandem walk is the kind of bullshit I think I should get to do without. It would be somewhat understandable if I were an even mildly educational case, but I'm not.

February 7, 2015

My Care Plan

Day 1: Rock on ✓
Day 2: Keep on Rockin'✓
Day 3: Rok Harder ✓
Days 4,5: Rock till you drop
Day 6: Rock Out

✓

J's care plan - implemented.

February 7, 2015

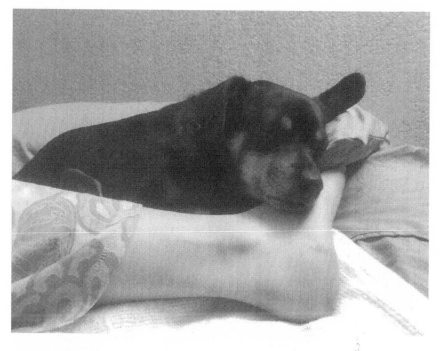

Cleo says "welcome home."

February 16, 2015

Whoopsidaisy!

It turns out that I have cancer and am going through chemo - I nearly forgot! That was until I was readmitted to the hospital last night with a fever, tachycardia, borderline blood pressure, and a white count (not to mention a hematocrit of 20 and platelets of 27 but presumably those are just "normal" mid-cycle labs). Fortunately I am not neutropenic but they admitted me since I met SIRS criteria and I was started on broad-spectrum antibiotics. They're keeping me for a 2nd night even though temperature, heart rate, and blood pressure are back to normal but my WBC bumped to 15 today and it hasn't yet been 24 hours on the cultures yet.

I feel remarkably well and am fairly asymptomatic. Yesterday I felt pretty good in the morning, even did some yard work, but then was tired and took a nap which was a little unusual. But what really concerned me was that when I woke up from my nap I didn't have much of an appetite and I looked at, and then took a bite of, a piece of cherry pie and then realized that I wasn't that into it - that's when I knew that there was something horribly wrong! A little later I was chilled so took my temp, had a fever, called my oncologist, went to UCSF ED (fortunately it was not rush hour!), was admitted, and here we are.

All the peds stuff just moved out of the hospital a few weeks ago to the new hospital at Mission Bay and my room is a former pediatric ICU room and it is the most horrible hospital room I have ever seen! It is small, dark, hot, and cramped and has no windows or bathroom. J thinks that they send the short patients here because regular sized beds seem too large for the room. I feel terribly for every parent who has had to be in this room with a sick kid and I'm very glad that they have their snazzy new rooms at Mission Bay. Thanks Mr. Benioff!

Assuming my cultures are negative and nothing develops/worsens I will be discharged tomorrow morning and can go back to nearly forgetting that I'm in the middle of chemo.

February 17, 2015

Here's a thought

Leaving the hospital feeling better than I did when I got here - amazing! This is so much better than feeling great when I arrive and crappy when I'm discharged! Someone should figure out how they can do this routinely; I'm sure there is a fortune in it somewhere.

Cultures all negative so my sepsis (!) was either due to a virus that didn't show up on the viral panel and didn't progress to cause further symptoms or a bacteria without an obvious source that was either adequately treated with 36 hours of antibiotics (!!!) or is gonna act up again in the next day or two. It will be exciting to see what happens!

In the meantime, I've got a slice of cherry pie to get back to.

February 18, 2015

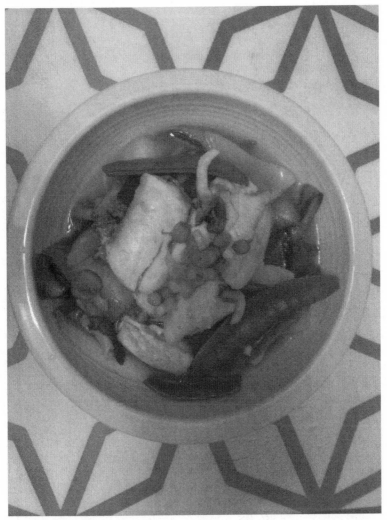

J's sepsis-treating lemongrass poached sea bass with bok
choy, snow peas, and oyster mushrooms.

It's working!

March 6, 2015

Update: 6 days in the hospital is still a really long time!

27.5 hours to go!

There has been a LOT of interest in my day-to-day so I thought I'd provide an overview. While not a complete accounting of my time here, I think it provides a nice taste. Twists and turns not included are the daily visit from the medicine team/hospitalist and oncology team and oncology NP (who is fucking awesome BTW and makes this whole thing significantly less painful), morning labs, q4hr vitals, a fun cocktail of PO meds, and a daily visit to the solarium - if free, daily visits from my mom, and J.

Hold on to your hats cause this is gonna be a wild ride.

Monday: call nursing station/wait for call from nursing station so that I don't come to the hospital until my bed is available - or, as happened this week, get call that bed is available earlier than ever (which would mean early discharge - yes!), drop everything (most notably the dog walk I was in the middle of), arrive at hospital 90 minutes later, find out that bed is no longer available, spend final 5 hours of freedom in hospital cafeteria waiting for bed to be available. Get into room at 7:30pm, blood draw (cause chemo can't

171

start until labs are back and it's faster to get stuck than to wait for them to access my port), cxr (cause boy those ports tend to move around a lot so it's best to check position once a month), other admission stuff, 4 hours of hydration after labs are back, premeds at 11:30 and 12, etoposide at 12:30am, ifosfamide/mesna at 1:30, mesna at 4:30 (repeat nightly).

Tuesday: start TID walks (4 cycles around the floor, alternate clockwise and counterclockwise just to keep things fresh), order banana from "room service," attempt to obtain 2 pieces of bread - request 2 pieces of bread, not successful, end up with 2 "triangles"

Wednesday: puff up, take a shower, change my clothes, read AAA magazine, 2nd attempt at obtaining 2 whole pieces of bread - ask for "4 triangles" - end up with 2

Thursday: diurese (always to the amazement of the medicine team, nearly prompting one of them to ask me if I'm measuring correctly! I wish they would ask so that I can finally confess that the challenge for me throughout my schooling was learning how to read volume in a graduated container.), read 1st of 3 issues of The Economist*, 3rd bread attempt - ask for "2 squares" - end up with 2 triangles

Friday: diurese, but stop recording my urine output (out of protest, for having cancer, and getting chemo, both of which are very stupid), take a shower, change my clothes, eat now ripe banana, read 2nd issue of the The Economist*, 4th bread attempt - ask for "twice the normal amount, the amount of bread traditionally used to make a standard sandwich" - success!

Saturday: read 3rd issue of The Economist*, watch the clock…

*Referred to in some circles as "US Weekly"

March 7, 2015

Thanks MLB!

What a glorious afternoon for a Giants spring training game broadcast! 135 minutes to go on infusion, 8th inning.

March 9, 2015

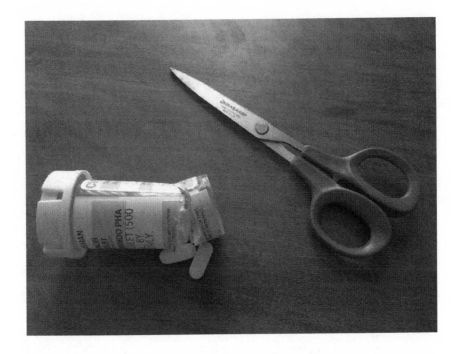

Frustrated? Me?

What makes you say that?

March 23, 2015

Busy week!

PET scan today, meet with pancreas surgeon on Wednesday, meet with lung surgeon on Friday. Then we meet with oncologist at the end of next week so that he can "bat cleanup." That was his second baseball analogy - the other one was that he said that he was "swinging for the fences" in terms of my treatment plan. I enjoyed them both!

March 28, 2015

The surgeons have spoken

Looks like I'm gonna have surgery. Probably start with a distal pancreatectomy and splenectomy in the next few weeks and assuming the recovery goes well lung surgery about a month later. I felt like I was in some sort of "flat affect-off" when I met with the pancreas surgeon and chief resident. I wanted to tell them that their suggestion to remove most of my pancreas and all of my spleen was not very dynamic.

The lung surgery will either be a wedge resection, or a lobectomy (more likely) and either VATS or mini-thoracotomy (more likely) and will either involve some repair of the vena cava or not (more likely as he thinks that there is a plane separating it from the tumor) but they won't know until they are in there. The surgeons still need to talk to each other, and I need to do some preop stuff (PFTs, echo, etc.), so

I do not yet have a start date. I meet with my oncologist in a few days and hope to have a better sense of specifics by that time. I am really hoping he no longer thinks I should do chemo after surgery. I would love to be done with chemo.

I have the PET results but have not heard what my oncologist thinks of them. There is reduced metabolic activity in all 4 lesions though not as significant a reduction as last time. The bone lesions are slightly larger but their metabolic activity is below background which seems like a good thing to me.

I discovered how deconditioned I am when I tried to use a rake today. Holy shit I was exhausted after two swipes! Clearly the moral is that I shouldn't try to use a rake.

April 4, 2015

Scheduled!

My distal pancreas (and spleen) and I will be parting ways the week of April 13th, exact date TBD.

I nearly forgot to mention that when I asked the lung surgeon what he thought surgery would buy me, he replied that his plan was that they would "keep tinkering" with me until I died of something else.

LMFAO!

April 7, 2015

Depressing

Since I've tried to keep this blog focused on the fun aspects of cancer I may have neglected to mention some of the sad realities. For instance, my limp. I've had it for about a year and it seems clear, 5 months after xrt, that it's not going anywhere. Fortunately my leg only hurts when I put weight on it which is easy to avoid by doing absolutely nothing. At least I never have to worry about my narcotics supply running low since I'm pretty sure "bone pain from cancer" gets you all you want. And it only takes a whiff of narcotics to make a big difference. But that same whiff usually leaves me face down on the bed in a spinning room. I realize that will get better but it still doesn't seem compatible with driving or being a clinician or anything else that requires being alert or having hand eye coordination. I've decided to put up with all this for now but J has agreed that if it gets to the point where it affects my footwear it will be perfectly understandable if I decide to give up on life.

April 19, 2015

POD 3 and pain musings

The surgery went well, no complications and they were able to do it laparoscopically although one of the wound sites is probably 4″ long because the tumor was softball sized (yikes!). They did also take my spleen and a bunch of lymph nodes. Doing pretty well - foley removed last night, advanced to full liquids today and hopefully more solid food tomorrow, epidural being weaned off today, able to walk around on my own, hope to go home late tomorrow or early Tuesday.

There was a major UCSF-caused, non-surgical clusterfuck that made POD 1 unnecessarily stressful and painful. The surgery was at Parnassus and J rented a place to stay for 4 nights within 5 minutes of Parnassus since it seemed like a bummer to have him far away (and potentially very far away depending on bridge traffic) especially if something unexpected happened. The morning after the surgery they told me that I was going to be transferred to Mission Bay, the new cancer hospital, that day, because that's where my surgery attending spends most of his time. They told me that transferring was mandatory and that it would definitely happen that day. So J gave up his rental (the whole issue of nobody even telling me I might be transferred is infuriating as we never would have gotten the rental but those issues I'm raising with my contact in the Patient Relations Dept!). Then later that day they said I wouldn't be transferred as there was no bed available! At that point I asked to at least be moved out of the incredibly shitty room I was in - which was basically 3 walls of curtains in a larger room with 3 other patients - no privacy, hot, noisy, no window, barely even room for a chair - since I had been there for more than a day. They call that a "semi-private" room which I think is some pretty funny propaganda since it is far worse than a normal 2 person room. Around 10pm there was a bed available at Mission Bay so paramedics showed up to transfer me. But the company didn't send critical care transport which was needed because of my epidural! So around 1am I was finally transferred to Mission Bay where I have a lovely, quiet, good-sized, private room with an awesome view (of the Bay Bridge) and everything is much, much better!

I think related to all that clusterfucking, I had a 3 hour period Friday evening when I was in a lot of pain and it took a while to get past it despite taking a quantity of narcotics that J found disturbing (he told me not to worry if a camera crew shows up and says they are doing a documentary about opiate use, it's not for the show "Intervention."). J thinks that I'm stoic and have a high pain tolerance - I don't know that either of those things are true but i am probably not as good as I could be about taking pain meds to keep me out of pain. But Friday night I was hitting that epidural button every 15 minutes, using 0.4mg hydromorphine boluses to get over the tough spots, and downed a few 5mg ocycodones, while they went up on my epidural basal rate. I thought I was dosing myself quite intelligently! Though it shouldn't have taken so long for me to get it under control. I have no doubt that the physical and psychological distress associated with the clusterfuck was a major contributor to this severe pain cause other than that episode my pain control has been quite good.

Today the plan was to wean me off the epidural and switch me to prn opiates which goes against everything I've ever learned about pain control. So instead I asked them to calculate my 24hr opiate use and they are putting me on 50% of that dose as standing. How is that not they way they always do things? I can't imagine going from 60 morphine equivalents to just prn meds!

But now, all good, hopefully recovery will continue on schedule and I can track down the pathologist cause I want to see my tumor!

April 20, 2015

POD 4 and lessons learned

1. It really hurts when they slice your belly open and remove a bunch of things.
2. Epidurals can provide a lot of pain control.
3. It doesn't take much (well, see #1, above) to go from a spinning room after 1 vicodin to taking shitloads of oxycodone with little effect.

I can't imagine that they will discharge me today given how many PRNs I am still taking, but I also thought there was no chance that mass in my lung was malignant!

Developing a 5-o'clock eyebrow shadow. It's very nice! Nothing on the head yet, but I don't mind, because if I weren't bald would the case manager have walked into my hospital room and asked if I was Mr. Rachel Roisman? I had fun with that. I realize it's not really fair to her, she works in a hospital, on a cancer service, she has probably never seen a bald woman before.

April 20, 2015

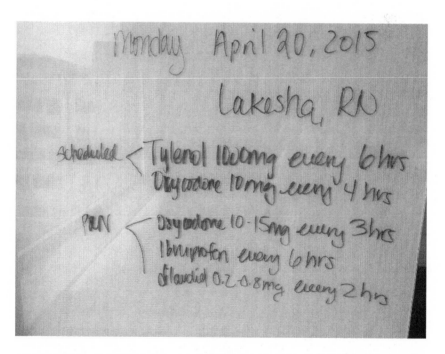

My pain med. regimen!

But it seems to be working, hopefully home tomorrow.

April 23, 2015

Home!

And I highly recommend it.

Actually, I got home on Tuesday but have been so happy to be here I have been remiss in my blogging. My appetite is picking up and I ate some pretty real food yesterday. The day I left the surgeon asked me an absurd question in an attempt to gauge my appetite - "did you eat more than half, or less than half, of your dinner?" Uhm, I ate all of my dinner, which was about 8oz of cream of wheat. How many times do you have to ask the question that way, and not get the information you need, before you realize that it's a ridiculous question?

Since J didn't think my plan to let cancer take its course if the hip pain starts interfering with my footwear was nearly as funny as I did, I decided to make up for it by getting a cane while I was in the hospital. I certainly don't need it all the time but on the bad days it will be pretty handy. Although the whole concept of needing a cane is uber depressing, I like the aesthetic of walking around with a cane and non-sensible shoes.

Say what you will about evidenced based medicine, but it's hard to beat having had someone cut me open and remove a softball-sized chunk of tumor cells. Next stop, the lungs, I assume late May/early Juneish.

April 29, 2015

Here we go again!

Lung surgery scheduled for May 28th. I hope I am not jinxing myself but It should be "easier" than the pancreas surgery with hopefully a slightly shorter hospital stay. Though the size of the pancreas tumor, which was not super well-determined by the PET/CT, makes me worried the lung lesion is also larger than expected and they won't be able to get it out without spreading my ribs. I won't know until after that if chemo is recommended though I am really hoping the answer is "no." Hard to imagine what I'll do with myself once this is all over.

The path report confirms that I have mesenchymal chondrosarcoma! Whew - what a relief! The pancreas tumor was 9.5 x 8.5 x 7.6 cm and weighed nearly 9 oz - holy shit! With all this space now available in my LUQ I feel as if I should start storing stuff there. Like doughnuts, I'm thinking doughnuts. The 11 lymph nodes were negative though I wasn't under the impression anyone ever thought they'd be anything other than negative. I've been in touch with the pathologist and he's willing to show me the specimens so I plan to go in sometime next week.

My recovery is going pretty well. I'm off the narcs and interested in eating though the referred shoulder pain I get when I eat limits my intake. I've been going for a little walk each day and can even sleep on my side again! But I sneezed for the first time yesterday and that was not fun. I've also had to limit my access to humor since laughing is still quite painful.

Eyebrows and eyelashes are now visible! They are more pronounced on the right than on the left. Is this because I spent too much time lying on my left side and all the chemo flowed downhill???

I saw the "other" way people deal with cancer yesterday - a black Mustang with a pink racing stripe and pink breast cancer ribbon emblazoned on the side, a license plate that translated to "Life is Good," AND a "Life is Good" license plate holder. Geez, celebrate life much? Well, it takes all kinds.

May 6, 2015

I touched my tumor

and I liked it!

Well, ceteris paribus, I'd rather not have a tumor but if I'm gonna have one it's nice to be able to touch it because a)it's interesting and b)it means it's not inside me. A pathology resident and fellow kindly took the time to show me my gross specimen and go over the slides with me. The tumor is neatly encapsulated and super firm in the middle where it is calcified.

Photos below for those who are not squeamish about this sort of thing.

Actually, the photos are below regardless. J thinks it is in poor taste but I certainly don't mean to offend, I just think it's very interesting.

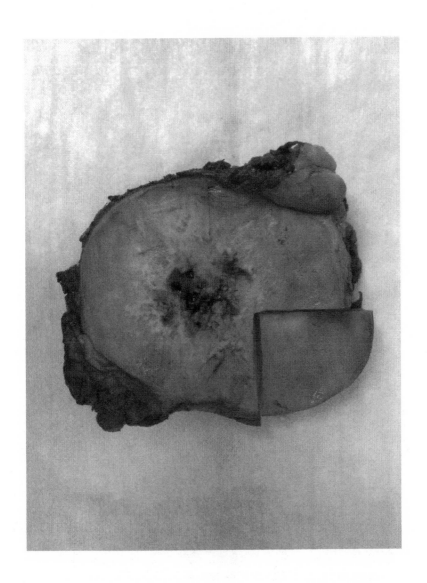

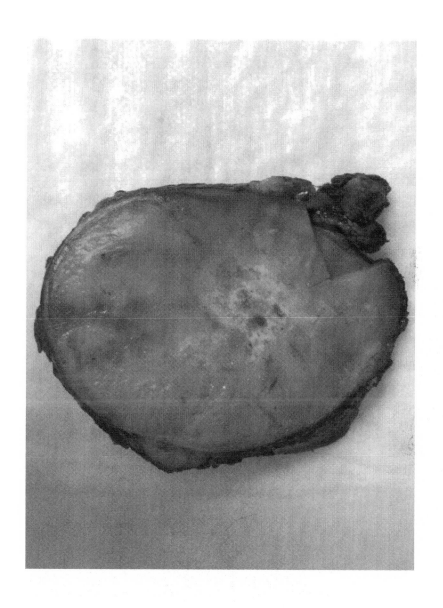

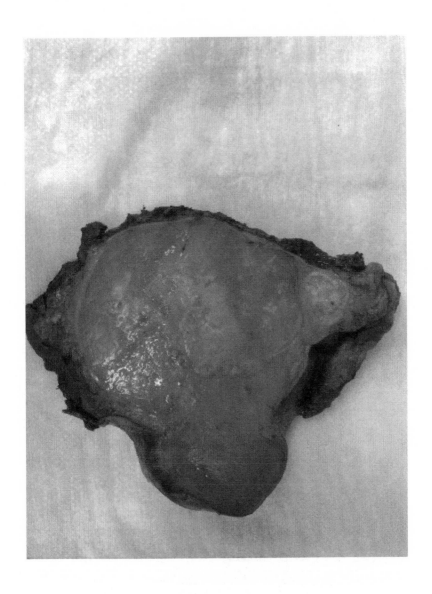

May 31, 2015

I peed in a toilet!

Baby steps.

POD 3 and doing fairly well. I never thought I would miss
the freedom I had when when I was tethered to an IV pole 24
hours a day for chemo, but in comparison it's far better than
being hooked up to 2 chest tubes, an epidural, 2 IVs, an
arterial line, a cardiac monitor, oxygen, and a foley catheter -
and being told that I should walk around a lot! I am now
down to one chest tube, the epidural, one IV, and the cardiac
monitor. I am supposed to use the oxygen, as long as I have
the epidural, but it doesn't even reach if I'm not in bed and I
usually forget when I'm in bed. J chided me and said that he
also likes to pick and choose the doctors suggestions he wants
to follow (which is totally true for him and super annoying!)
but I told him that the difference is that I'm not sitting here
complaining of shortness of breath *and* not using my oxygen.
I'm not saying he does that sort of thing…but he does. Maybe
I'll put the oxygen on…

I'm still a little fuzzy on the details of the surgery but the
surgeon thought it was 50-50 going in that he could do VATS
vs. a thoracotomy (and wedge resection vs. lobectomy) but it
turned out that the mass was bigger than expected and up
against all sorts of important things so they had to do the full
thoractomy and lobectomy to get everything out. The surgeon
had that little smile on his face when he told me what
happened, the one that says, "I was surprised that your
surgery was trickier than expected and it was a super fun

surprise cause I love the challenge of dissecting tumor away from important structures." You know the look. J was thrilled - oh, sure, of course with the fact that the surgery went well - but with the longer surgery. When they said VATS could be 30 minutes J said "oh no, I was really hoping to be able to get some sleep!" I told him that he was a horrible, horrible person.

Apparently the first thing I said to J when I woke up was "Did I miss any good stories? Did anything really funny happen?" At least I am true to myself when I'm completely zonked. I spent a night in the ICU, standard for a lobectomy, and the ICU attending was a former co-resident of mine which was far more nice than incredibly odd. I planned to be a really difficult patient and do things like demand blood transfusions for low-normal hematocrits but I never got around to it. Yesterday I moved out of the ICU to a regular floor where I have a lovely little single room. I am hoping that they can remove the other chest tube today, which would mean the epidural comes out too, and I might be able to go home tomorrow!!!

June 1, 2015

Heading home!

That's the plan, anyway. The second chest tube was removed yesterday; score one for chest tube in the chest tube vs. abdominal tube contest - waaaay faster, easier, and less painful than having the JP drain removed. The epidural just

190

came out; pain is still an issue but I think I can manage it at home. I enjoyed how much pain the pain team caused by the manner in which they removed the epidural dressing; it's that sort of absurdity that makes this blog possible.

I used to think it was really sad when I saw patients with their little butts hanging out of their gowns - a seemingly complete loss of self respect - and while I certainly can't presume to know their reasons for tolerating it, it now seems perfectly reasonable to me. Mostly I really don't give a shit. I guess after you've had people's hands all over the inside of your body there isn't much mystery that seems necessary to try to keep. If I didn't think it would risk a "Code Green" I'd be perfectly happy doing this postop thing completely naked so as to make things easier - easier to move around without having to thread tubing in and around my gown, easier than having to change gowns each time my dressing soaked through, easier than having to disrobe so someone can listen to my lungs, or look at my incision site, or give me some sq heparin. The only problem with doing this half-way (neither fulled en- or disrobed) is that I imagine anybody who catches a glimpse of my backside is going to be saddened by my seemingly complete loss of self respect and not realize that it actually represents a complete loss of giving a shit.

Ah, the insight that being a doctor with cancer brings. It's such a beautiful thing.

June 3, 2015

Holy shit!

I take back any and every mean thing I have ever said about epidurals. If I had an epidural in, and better use of the right side of my body, I would write "I will not badmouth epidurals" 100 times on a blackboard to prove my sincerity. It just goes to prove that you don't know what you've got till it's gone. Don't know what it is I did so wrong. Now I know what I got it's just this song and it ain't easy to get back takes so long.

Unfortunately, there's a wide gap between the amount of pain meds I take and the amount of pain meds I need, and that gap is filled with nausea. I kind of thought that didn't happen and I'd be able to tolerate as much as I needed! Fortunately hot packs do wonders. More fortunately, these things tend to heal and I am very slowly moving in the right direction. But this is the most dysfunctional I've been from all this treatment. Fortunately, J is there to laugh at me when I get stuck in a weird position in bed that I can't get out of on my own. He does also lift me up, but he likes to do the laughing part first.

June 10, 2015

More path!

The path resident sent me these photos of the microscopic H&E (hematoxylin and eosin) stain of the pancreas tumor so I thought I'd share them. I haven't yet tried to see the lung path because I'm not mobile enough but I hope to get to see them in the next few weeks.

{At one point there were pictures included below in the original blog but they are no longer available, probably removed by Rachel for some reason so only the tags are included now}

Biphasic Tumor I

4x magnification

10x

20x

Biphasic Tumor II 20x

40x

Biphasic Tumor III 10x

20x

Biphasic Tumor IV 4x

10x

Chondroid Area 20x

Fibrous Area 4x

10x

20x

Spindled Area 10x

20x

Tumor and normal pancreas 4x

Tumor with hemangiopericytomatous vessels 4x

10x

June 12, 2015

Mission accomplished!

That's what the thoracic surgeon said - and I like it! I had my 2 week postop visit today and he thinks it's good that they got the tumor out when they did, and he thinks my recovery is going well. I was a bit worried about the "focally present at inked resection margin" comment in the path report but the surgeon said the tumor was not transected and there was a clear, but very flimsy, plane of fat between the tumor and all the good stuff. The tumor was not invading, or difficult to separate from, the surrounding tissue. From his perspective,

195

I'd get lung CTs every 3 months for the next year and then every 6 months after that, assuming nothing new shows up. But really the question is what my oncologist thinks should be done and I won't know his plan for another 2 weeks.

The only really "awesome" thing about going to these appointments is the side trip to the nearby French bakery. I told J to just get a few things since I didn't want to feel pressured to eat an insane number of pastries in the next day or two or deal with the heartache of letting excellent pastries go past their prime. I think we had a failure to communicate because he came back with 6 pastries, 2 cookies, and a bag of snazzy granola! I probably shouldn't expect him to show restraint if I send him to buy pastries proximate to a doctor's appt that is more than 50% related to my having cancer.

June 19, 2015

Hirsute

That's what J said I am becoming. I told him that was one of the worst things ever said to a woman while her face was being touched. He said "chill out, Teen Wolf" and then started singing Werewolves of London. I told him he is the worst spouse of a woman with cancer, ever.

June 26, 2015

Reprieve!

We met with my oncologist yesterday and he is very pleased with how the treatment has gone and how I've responded to it (he said that I can really take a punch!) so no more chemo for now!!! The plan is another scan early August and if things are stable (nothing growing, nothing new) then scans every 3 months for a while. So now all I have to do is get over this thoracotomy, and I'm working on that.

By the way, my hip has been much better of late and I'm not limping nearly as much as I was before. My dad's theory, which I think is a pretty good one, is that the bone lesions saw what happened to the lung and pancreas lesions and realized that they needed to lay low for a while or they are gonna get fucked up.

August 6, 2015

Not the best news ever...

though not exactly the worst either.

I had CT chest/abd/pelvis and MRI abdomen (still not clear to me why that was ordered, or why it was ordered by the thoracic surgeon, maybe he is trying to branch out) and there are 3 tiny (6mm) spots in the abdomen/pelvis that are definitely not clearly mets, but they could be. My oncologist is not freaked out so I've decided that I'm not either, but obviously I would have preferred an "all clear." One of the spots is fairly superficial so they'll try an ultrasound-guided biopsy in a week and then it will be several more days before the results are available.

I anticipate that household ice cream and pastry expenditures will increase significantly over the next 10 days.

The chest CT report included a comment about a wedge resection of a RLL nodule - which, for the record, never happened. I've decided that I'm going to invent a device that will non-invasively scan parts of the body and provide an accurate image of what is inside - I'm gonna be a billionaire.

August 14, 2015

Biopsy complete

I had the biopsy done yesterday - the good news is that they were able to biopsy both superficial lesions (the 3rd lesion is in the splenic fossa so nobody is getting there easily) so we'll know what both of them are. The bad news is that I had lesions to biopsy. The biopsy itself was pretty easy and the pathologist was in the room and he analyzed the samples to make sure enough cells were obtained so that dramatically improves the chances that we'll have an answer. The results will take several days so now we just try to distract ourselves while awaiting a phone call.

Ice cream futures remain a good investment opportunity.

August 20, 2015

Waiting...

Despite the fact that the pathologist who was present at the biopsy told me to expect results by mid-week, now I'm being told that actually it normally takes 10-14 days for results.

Not as if the results dramatically impact my immediate future or anything.

August 26, 2015

ugh.

Both spots are malignant. My oncologist thinks I should probably do more chemo but he's going to discuss me at tumor board later this week. He doesn't think that I should do the chemo regimen I just did and I'm going to have some tumor typing done to see if there is a specific target. Of course this will probably take a few weeks to get straightened out. Once he has a suggestion we plan to have a discussion about likely benefits cause I don't want to do more chemo just for the sake of doing more chemo - as fun as it is. I've really been enjoying having hair - I'm nearly stylish at this point. Obviously J and I are both devastated. We had a few months of very future-oriented thinking which now seems rather premature.

August 26, 2015

Cupcakes

I always buy the mini ones, even though the flavors are more limited. They are just so cute, and tasty. I tend to like mini most things - except bagels, mini bagels are absurd as they cannot support smoked fish. And mini metastases, while probably better than regular sized ones, I still don't like them very much.

We had mediocre BBQ tonight - never again - I do not have time for this shit.

August 29, 2015

{Link to the song "Limbo Rock" by Chubby Checker *was embedded here}*

They weren't able to discuss me at tumor board this week so I have to wait until next week. But the tumor sequencing blood test results won't be back for a few weeks so I don't expect tumor board to be that useful cause they'll probably just say something like "we should wait for the tumor sequencing results." In the meantime, I'm mostly focused on wondering what it's gonna be like when this tumor in my gluteal muscles becomes "softball-sized" and I can't wear pants or sit down anymore. That seems like a reasonable thing to focus on especially given the alternative which is wondering what it's gonna be like when the paraspinal tumor becomes "softball-sized."

September 5, 2015

Hang on to your sweatpants...

Finally got to talk to my oncologist yesterday and he said I was discussed at tumor board and his recommendation is radiation to the 3 new spots and then more chemo. He doesn't know which chemo, though more of the inpatient regimen is likely, and he doesn't know for how long. He'll figure that out in the next few weeks. So a very, very tentative schedule is 3 weeks of radiation in September, a month off to recover, chemo starting in November. No part of this seems "good," but at least I have some idea what the next few months might hold.

September 14, 2015

And the hits just keep on coming.

Last week my right leg started hurting - for the first time ever. As you may recall, I've got a spot in my femur (neck) on that side and it was radiated last November. Even though it has always been the left side (acetabulum) that has been painful, the right side is more of an issue because the femur is weight-bearing and a pathologic fracture will really fuck with my life. Needless to say, getting pain on that side was not a happy development. I think it may have been because I walked up some stairs (it was imaged, there is no fracture), something I don't normally encounter in my one-story craftsman existence. So today I took the fucking elevator. This is really starting to get depressing.

October 6, 2015

WTF???

Amazing how often that is an appropriate header.

What follows are separate conversations I've had with my oncologist (ONC), radiation oncologist (RADONC), and the surgeon who did my splenectomy/distal pancreatectomy (SURG). I had all of these conversations separately but am presenting them in chronological order so you can appreciate how insanely frustrating this is! I've condensed them into one blog post for your reading pleasure but it would be a more accurate representation of my experience if I spread these out over the 6+ weeks it has been since I got the biopsy results. Italicized comments represent my takeaway after each visit/phone conversation.

ONC: You have 3 new mets (2 superficial, 1 abdominal in the area formerly known as "spleen"). The surgeon, radiation oncologist, and I spoke at tumor board. You should have radiation to the 3 spots and then chemo.

_____[*ugh, more chemo, that sucks, radiation doesn't seem that bad*]_____

RADONC: Sure, I can radiate the 3 lesions. Radiation could give you 2 2.5cm areas of your skin that are sunburned. Maybe you should have the 2 superficial ones removed surgically? I discussed this with the surgeon and he said he can remove them.

ME: As an outpatient procedure with some local anesthesia or am I gonna be intubated in the OR?

RADONC: I didn't ask him that

ME: Uhm, isn't that kind of the only thing that matters? Correct me if I'm wrong, but you're suggesting I consider undergoing general anesthesia to avoid the pain and suffering associated with two small sunburns?????

RADONC: You should ask him that. By the way, I spoke with the oncologist yesterday, and he doesn't think you necessarily need to do chemo after radiation

ME: Hmm, that's not what he told me last week.

RADONC: Well, he does change his mind sometimes.

_____[*Can't figure out what he's not telling me to even suggest surgery is preferable to radiation. Regardless - yay - may not need chemo!*]_____

RADONC: I'm not sure I can radiate the abdominal lesion - it is so small I can't be sure that I can target it - I need to discuss this with the radiologists.

____[*Hmm, ok, well, since the abdominal lesion is the most unpleasant to radiate - more risks and side effects - that doesn't seem so bad if he can't radiate it.*]_____

ONC: I spoke to the surgeon and he doesn't think surgery is a good idea on the superficial lesions - could be a lot of digging around, hard to get clean margins, might need a flap to close, recovery could be rough. If all 3 lesions can be radiated then you should do that and we will follow closely with another scan in 2-3 months. If the abdominal lesion can't be radiated then radiate the other two and then do chemo and we will follow the abdominal lesion to see how it responds to chemo. So you will do 2-6 months of chemo, depending on the response.

ME: I'm not that excited about chemo. If the abdominal lesion is too small to radiate now, isn't the "good news" that it will keep growing and then it can be radiated?

ONC: That is one way of looking at it. It wouldn't be unreasonable if you decided not to do chemo now.

_____[*Oh, disregard earlier comment, now I better hope they can radiate the abdominal lesion so that chemo isn't even on the table. If he can't radiate the abdominal lesion, I might opt against chemo anyway but it would be easier if I didn't feel like I was going against my oncologist's advice.*]_____

SURG: Hi, I'm thinking we should do surgery to remove the two superficial lesions. This can be done as an outpatient with local anesthesia and conscious sedation, it will probably take 30 minutes.

ME: What about the can't get clean margins/might need to dig around a lot/could need a skin flap/rough recovery?

SURG: No, none of that.

ME: And this is better than radiation?

SURG: Always better to get it out than radiate.

ME: And what about the abdominal lesion?

SURG: I'm not sure about that - just follow it with scans.

ME: Uhm, ok

__[*Shit, so now I should have surgery??? Does my oncologist even know that the surgeon is now saying the exact opposite of what my oncologist told me less than a week ago?*]___

This all happened AFTER I was discussed at tumor board! I sure as fuck am not doing more chemo in the absence of a more clear recommendation that it might be worthwhile. Not sure what to do about the surgery...

October 9, 2015

I'll see your paraspinal lesion and raise you a skull met.

Alternate title: Fuuuuuuucccccccckkkkkkk me

Yep, the shit has officially hit the fan. I've been having headaches over the past week and yesterday noticed some swelling in the right temporal area so I went to the ED, more concerned about some insidious infection since skull mets don't develop overnight, and a CT scan revealed a 3x3cm mass in the right greater sphenoid wing and squamous temporal bone. The mass is intra and extracranial but I'm not having neuro symptoms and there is no mass effect or other obvious impact on the brain. The mass was not there on the PET scan done in March but it was present on the mid-September PET scan it just wasn't noticed because the brain metabolic activity makes it difficult to see anything going on in that area. It was about the same size in September. I always knew that skull mets were an option and I wondered how those would be discovered since the PET scan isn't a good way to detect them. Looks like I was right to worry about that. My oncologist was called with the results but I haven't spoken with him yet. I suspect the next step is radiation and then chemo. So the plan that was finally settled 2 days ago (surgery to remove the 2 superficial mets, follow the abdominal lesion) is now out the window. And while I wasn't planning on doing chemo after surgery, if he recommends it now I'd probably do it just because I think chemo is preferable to more, or bigger, mets in the neighborhood of the brain.

It is amazing how much more, and persistently, painful these headaches are now that I know what's causing them. When I thought they were because I was stressed or tired or not drinking enough water or coffee they were pretty mild.

Having the ED resident conduct a neuro exam on me reminded me of being in that same ED 10 years ago and having to do a neuro exam on a neurologist with a Bell's Palsy who decided to pimp me during the exam. That was fun. In honor of that experience I opted to point out to the resident that he missed CN XI and XII. My life now seems so limited I feel I have to take advantage of every opportunity to be douchey to trainees.

October 17, 2015

Cancer in your head? I thought you said there's a dancer in the shed!

Apparently I am the only one who thinks this is a big deal! After not hearing from my oncologist in 4 days (yes, 2 weekend days included) I called his cell (something I reserve for urgent issues, you know, like being told you have cancer in your skull) and he seemed surprised by the sense of urgency in my voice. Only after the phone call did he order the MRI (which I had the next day) and talk to radiation oncology (apparently I was supposed to contact them myself, but I thought he was going to refer me to neuro radonc, you know, because of the cancer in the skull).

Anyway, I saw radonc yesterday, and he's not convinced xrt is the way to go (might cause some lasting headaches that need to be treated with steroids or surgery - something about necrosis - a word I love to hear in conjunction with the term "brain cells," could impact my vision, not likely to shrink the lesion, may not control the lesion). He already discussed my case with neurosurgery and they seem to think surgery makes sense (I am shocked, shocked, to find that the surgeons think they should do surgery!). I have an appt with them on Tuesday.

The terrible sounding piece of news - which I've decided is not much worse than what the news already was - mostly because I still need to be able to get out of bed in the morning

- is that the MRI showed extension into the brain parenchyma (8mm). The whole lesion is pretty fucking big - an untrained monkey could point it out on the scan - it's about 4x3cm in total with 2x3cm mass inside the skull and a similar sized mass outside the skull. I guess we'll see what the surgeons say. If this is a very straightforward procedure for them, then I'll consider it. But if there's anything tricky or risky about it I can't imagine wanting to take those chances.

Insert witty sign-off here...

October 20, 2015

"No, no, we take the tumor, leave the brain behind."

I guess if you're gonna have someone operate on your head, the best you can hope for is that they think of the surgery as so straightforward as to be dull. We met with the neurosurgeon today who seemed pretty unimpressed with the whole situation. He said the surgery will take 4-5 hours, and I got the impression the 5 hours would be if he fell asleep in the middle of it because it was so fucking boring. I should be in the hospital for about 3 nights which would be shorter than the stay for my other operations. And he doesn't expect any cosmetic or neurologic defects afterward. The schedule is TBD but most likely next week.

October 21, 2015

And so it goes

Monday afternoon my skull tumor and I will part ways - hopefully. If it's gotta happen, and apparently it does, I'm glad to have it happen sooner rather than later.

Still struggling to come up with a hilarious zinger.

October 22, 2015

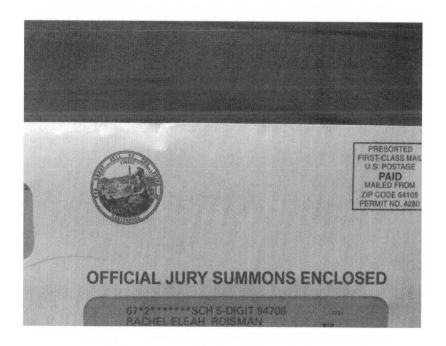

File under "completely fucking absurd."

Or, "do you mind if my craniotomy wound gets blood on your jury box?"

November 1, 2015

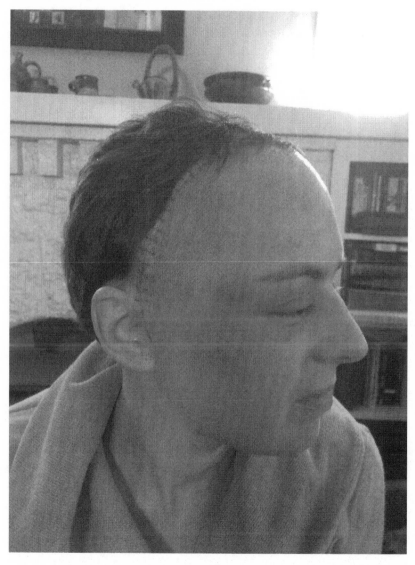

In case you thought I was completely fucking around about having my skull cracked open 6 days ago, here's a little visual proof. The sutures run over the top of my head, ear to ear. The left side of my face looks fairly normal but the swelling on the right side is still pretty freaky looking. Today was the first day that my right eye wasn't swollen shut when I woke up so that is progress!

It is remarkable how little pain there is - I haven't had any pain medicine since POD 2! The only discomfort is from the edema. I am still on steroids as part of a long taper to reduce the edema. And I'll be off seizure prophylactic medication in another day or two. Overall I'm doing pretty well. I certainly would not have guessed that this would have been the "easiest" of the three surgeries. The postop nausea/vomiting was the worst with this surgery but I think that's just because the anesthesiologists didn't bother to do whatever they did the first 2 times that worked so well.

I definitely feel as if I've had more than my fair share of major surgery (and in only 6 months!); I'm pretty ready to be done with this shit.

November 3, 2015

Good to know

Steroids make me really fucking anxious! It's a lovely combo of drunk/high fuzzy-headedness, with intermittent nausea, and without the fun parts, layered on a jittery, sleepless base of anxiety. So much for my plan to use steroids to help me suck the marrow out of life. Well, speaking of marrow…they do help the appetite. And here I was hoping I could add a nice auto-immune disorder to my repertoire just so I would have an excuse to stay on them longer. Where's all the fun I was promised??? Taper will finish in a few days - cannot happen soon enough.

November 13, 2015

Not psychotic!

It occurred to me that I should post some sort of update lest my readers think that I had a steroid-induced psychotic break. Steroids are done, stitches are out, swelling is greatly diminished, hairline still looks incredibly freaky prompting the wearing of a hat while in public, and will be able to drive next week. I'm gonna have this partial botox look (can't raise my right eyebrow, no wrinkles on the right side of my forehead) for a few months, but that is surprisingly low on my list of concerns. And besides, it just makes my left eyebrow raising that much more dramatic and meaningful. If only I could find some things about which to be wry and cynical so I can put that skill to good use…where's a crappy situation when you need one???

I've got follow-up scans next week and see my oncologist the following week to find out what unpleasant chemo regimen he recommends (Happy Thanksgiving!). I am also hoping that we can have a bit of a big picture discussion about what is the fucking point of doing more chemo since the last chemo I did, which was deemed useful at the time (based on scan results), didn't exactly prevent 3+ new mets (jury is out on whether the one in the splenic fossa is actually a met since it wasn't metabolically active on the PET) developing (including a super fun one in my skull) within a few months of my stopping it. On the other hand, I'd really like to avoid having another met to my skull, or another similarly unpleasant locale, so it wouldn't take a lot for him to convince me that it's worth trying. At least with chemo it can always be stopped at any point.

I got the results from the tumor sequencing (Guardant360 - blood, Foundation One - tissue) and unfortunately there is nothing "actionable." I was really hoping that the tumor had some sort of anti-milkshake genetic mutation so that the relevant targeted therapy would be to drink a lot of milkshakes.

Damn it!

When does all the good stuff related to having metastatic bone cancer start happening???

November 29, 2015

More mets

Yeah, sorry, no good news to report. My most recent scan showed that the 2 superficial lesions are larger (1-2cm) and there are 3 new mets (2 1cm pleural nodules and a 3cm cardiophrenic mass). My oncologist was unpleasantly surprised that there have been so many new lesions since I stopped chemo about 6 months ago, and that they are growing relatively rapidly. Though the "good" news is that growing more rapidly means chemo might work better - we found that swimming at the bottom of the "silver lining" barrel along with "I probably don't need to worry about my internal medicine board recertification." His best guess as to why this cancer that hasn't produced any new lesions in 2 ½ years has become so prolific is that the postop environment with all of its excited little cells helped prompt tumor growth - which is not to say that it was a mistake to have surgery - it just is what it is. He suggests the same inpatient chemo regimen I did earlier this year since I had a "good" response to that chemo. But he acknowledges that this is a good time to start thinking about whether chemo is worthwhile. If I have anything less than an "extraordinary" response to 2 cycles of chemo ("extraordinary" in the pornographic, "know it when I see it" kind of way) then it's not worth continuing. There are a range of other options (outpt chemo, radiation to the cardiophrenic lesion which is the most problematic one since it doesn't have a lot of room to grow, some sort of experimental/clinical trialy option, do nothing). We are mulling things over and expect to make a decision mid-Decish.

Thanksgiving was not super thanks-oriented this year.

December 15, 2015

Two steps back from the brink?

I went to LA and met with an oncologist who pretty much just does sarcoma clinical trials. He has used a newer med (trabectedin) in 4-5 patients with mesenchymal cs with good results (reduced tumor size - and yes, the plural of anecdote IS evidence!) and it is less unpleasant than regular chemo so he suggested trying that twice (given as a 24 hour outpatient infusion once every 3-4 weeks). My regular oncologist thinks it's a reasonable approach so I'm going to try it. Next steps are a baseline PET scan, insurance "approval" (I'm sure my HMO will love to approve off-label use of a med by a physician outside my network!), and then 2 trips to LA over the next two months for the infusion. If a PET scan shows improvement then hopefully I can transition to getting the med in SF. They have been using the med as maintenance therapy in some patients with sarcoma - for 2+ years - since it "doesn't have any longterm effects."

Ha!

But, still, as much as I enjoyed being a teaching case for the med students, this option seems far preferable and well worth a try. The biggest problem is that if it sort of works I may actually have to take the boards next year. The best part is that maybe I can be part of a new indication for this drug (short brown-haired women aged 41-42 who like scones - good scones) so I can help extend the patent life and keep it from becoming generic for another 7+ years! Maybe I can become a spokesperson for the pharmaceutical company

("I'm not just a doctor, I'm a patient!") Surely there is an upcoming sarcoma conference in Fiji? Do you think they have any pens I can start using? How about a stuffed transcription factor I can use as a dog toy? Or a waterslide painted the color of the drug company and made out of marshmallows that is both a children's toy and a meal replacement?

Someone get me a rolling laptop bag and a platter of sandwiches, stat!

This shall be my legacy!

December 27, 2015

Well, that was fun.

Xmas Eve in the ED. I had this very difficult to localize, completely new, moderately severe, right-sided flank/upper abdominal pain for about 24 hours that was not going anywhere with heat, nsaids, or even oxycodone and after spending much of the day lying in bed it seemed like I should get checked out. It wasn't very crowded and for an ED visit it went fairly smoothly. Other than some pain-related hypertension my vitals were normal as were my labs and a bedside RUQ US. Since I'd just had a PET/CT and wasn't eager for another contrast CT that would only be useful if something had developed in the past week, everyone (ED MDs, radiologist, me) agreed that more scanning didn't seem useful and it was probably the cardiophrenic mass causing some irritation. And after a mg of hydromorphone I wasn't exactly feeling any pain any more. So I got home around 4am. Too bad I didn't get home around 3:50am as then I could have vomited in the house rather than in the car - still such a narcotic neophyte. Fortunately, the pain subsided and I haven't needed anything since the ED visit.

Tomorrow, supposedly, we are going to LA to start the trabectedin on Tuesday. There is still no answer from the insurance company - which actually appears to be the fault of the clinic rather than the insurance company - but at this point it doesn't seem like I can really wait around and let these things get bigger. Until I'm actually getting the meds I'm not convinced this is going to happen on Tuesday but that is the current plan.

December 29, 2015

Room Service Menu

Open Daily 7:00am to 8:00pm

Call 3-1111 to place order

Delivery within 60 minutes

Patients at Mission Bay have the option to place orders through their bedside tablet.

Our kitchen system and clerk knows your food allergies and prescribed diet from your health record. Patient's name, date of birth, and prescribed diet will be verified. Some items from the menu may be restricted according to the doctor's orders. There is no charge for this service for patients.

UCSF Medical Center
Nutrition & Food Services

Great little bistro in SF.

Back in, issues with my right eye, a little swelling, a little blurry vision, dash of discomfort, sprinkle of proptosis, came to ED for expedited MRI, prelim shows swelling at surgical site and around optic nerve, admitted for steroids (yay!) and expedited eval, more deets when I have them.

December 29, 2015

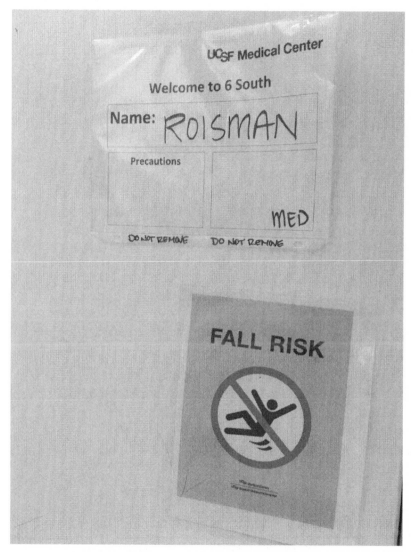

Really?????

Now they are just trying to hurt my feelings.
December 29, 2015

Don't nobody bring me...

That one is for you LFD!

But, sadly, they did, more bad news. I've got a new skull/head met, it's basically in the same spot as the old one. It's about 4cm with a necrotic center (delicious! Surgery isn't on the table but I did mean to ask if they could just jab a straw in there and suck it out. Not just any straw, obviously it would have to be sterile). It compresses the temporal lobe dura/parenchyma but isn't invading the parenchyma. It is also expanding into the orbit (in part because part of that back of orbit bone was removed) and it is causing mass effect on the lateral rectus muscle and is also getting into the muscles of mastication and the temporalis muscle. This was not present 6 weeks ago when I last had an MRI of my brain. This discovery was prompted by the observation, mostly by J, that the swelling that had been improving post-op had no long continued to improve and was in fact getting worse. And Sunday night I realized that my right eye was becoming proptotic. So I contacted neurosurgery and rad. onc. and they said go to the ED for an MRI since that's the only mildly efficient way of getting a scan in the middle of the holidays. If you call a nearly 10hr wait in a bed in the ED hallway "efficient."

Were I into twitter, the whole ED stay would have made for some great (albeit overly long) tweets.

- They just wheeled up demented/delirious woman who recently refused MRI to radiology for MRI - unmedicated - can't wait to see how long it takes for them to bring her back without MRI being done! Answer: 30 minutes. Transport person "she said she couldn't see so they sent her back." RN: "She always says things like that, that's why she needs the MRI!" Classic!

- Non-English speaking elderly woman in the room next to me calling for help - torn by desire to not be a terrible person but also curious to know how long this can go on before someone helps.

Just for the record, I did go for help.

- I overheard a nurse give report on a patient and describe the patient as not having an "intact sense of humor." J and I worked out that he'll pull the plug as soon as my sense of humor dips below a level 5. There is some concern because we haven't actually established the scale. Though at the very least that will be a hilarious way to go…"while Vegas had her at 1:100 going out on cancer, she actually went out over a tragic misunderstanding related to a misguided health care proxy arrangement and an unclearly logarithmic humor scale."

I was admitted overnight for an expedited workup and I was started on steroids and just got home tonight! I talked to neurosurgery, rad. onc. and oncology, and optho. The plan is xrt to the head lesions ASAP - in the next few days - and then trabectedin, which is arriving at UCSF next week (I will be the first UCSF patient! And my insurance approved it!). There is an outstanding issue as to how long I have to wait in between radiation and chemo but probably just a week or two. In the end, a remarkable coordination of care - which I think can be attributed to the awesome onc. NP who took care of me during my inpt chemo and does things like schedule appts mid-day so as to help us avoid bridge traffic and builds in extra time because she knows that the first time this med is given is going to take longer than normal. It did remind me of a famous inpatient note I once read about a patient with diffuse vascular disease who spent days and days hanging out in the hospital while the cardiologists and the nephrologists and the vascular surgeons and the interventional radiologists all couldn't agree about what should happen first. But that Janet Jackson does have really nice breasts.

I only expect about 6 people reading this to know wtf I'm talking about, but that's ok!

Oh yeah, so I didn't go to LA yesterday.

December 31, 2015

Scheduled!

Radiation starts Tuesday and will end the following Monday. No exact timing on chemo yet. In the meantime, the steroids have been reducing the swelling which is nice cause it makes me feel like something positive is going on. Also, I have not (yet) become psychotic and am mostly just wired. But jesus I am on some high dose steroids and this is going to continue through and after xrt for a while. The swelling wasn't that dramatic but now that it is going down it is more apparent that my face was a bit fucked up.

In case you were wondering if it complicates matters to have cancer recur in exactly the same spot where it was just removed - yes, it does! For one thing, with the bone they removed there was more room for the new lesion to grow before it became apparent to the naked eye AND of course I had some swelling and visual symptoms post-op and since they were gradually improving how the fuck was I supposed to notice when they gradually started to worsen? Fortunately J is very noticey and he started to comment, in a very sensitive way, to my fucked up face. As has been apparent from the start of all this, my subscription to the "common things being common" and "when you hear hoofbeats don't think of zebras" mantras hasn't been really helpful. "Why would I be freaked out, it's not likely that it's malignant" I fondly recall telling my new PCP when I needed an ASAP referral to pulmonary for evaluation of the recently discovered chest mass. Hilarious!

This sets aside the whole question, which I do plan to ask, about cancer showing up in the same spot 2 months later! Unless the temporal part of my skull has been aggressively advertising itself as a hospitable locale for cancer cells, it must be that there was something left that kept growing. It can't be common and I was told everything was removed. So I asked the neurosurgery resident, not expecting him to have an answer, and he said "well, it is at a microscopic level." To which I wanted to suggest that they do something during the surgery where they use an instrument that can detect things at a microscopic, even cellular, level to see if there is any cancer present not just in what they removed but on the edges of what is left. They could call it something like "edges free" so that everyone would know that they removed all the cancer! I wouldn't expect the surgeons to have to do this during the operation but perhaps the pathologists could come in and help out? They could use one of their fancy microscopes or something? Just an idea! I fear that I am an M+M (and no, not the delicious candy that melts in your mouth and not in your hands kind of way, more of the kind that apparently "rocked the nation" when shown on TV as part the Hopkins 24/7 series" http://articles.baltimoresun.com/2000-09-10/news/0009080268_1_mm-patient-care-surgeon). And I don't necessarily mean that something got fucked up, I just mean that in addition to this being a super crappy outcome is must also be a pretty unusual one. I'd like to attend that M+M...pretty sure they are not going to let me do that.

January 7, 2016

I am running out of ways to say that things just keep getting shittier and shittier and shittier...

I guess I was naive to expect that my 3rd trip to the ED in 10 days would have turned out well. But how much worse could it be than "hey, that skull met we removed 2 months ago is now back and bigger than it was before!"?

Hard to top that, but they got with me with the thing I knew, from day 1, was going to completely fuck me up once it started, reduced mobility. I've got my first pathological fracture! My left hip pain has been an issue since the beginning but about 6 months ago it got a lot better (which was 6 months after xrt) and my limp was much improved. Even though that lesion was the only one that caused pain, everyone was much more concerned about the right femur spot since that's a weight-bearing bone. But I only ever had pain on the right side once. The past few weeks the pain on the left has been worse - but just worse than it had been for a few months - not worse than it's been in the past. Sunday night, without anything in particular happening, it gradually got really, really worse. And whereas the pain is generally localized to the left groin, Sunday night the pain was hard to localize, throughout most of my left thigh, and severe despite the consumption of what I thought was a truly remarkable amount of pain medicine (in the past 3 years there have been about 5 occasions when I've needed the equivalent of 1-2 vicodin for hip/leg pain, between 9pm Sunday and 5am Monday morning I took 70mg of oxycodone and was still completely awake and had no reduction in my pain) - that was when it seemed like an ED visit might be needed. Since it was 7am on a workday, and I was in excruciating pain, a 90 minute rush-hour commute to UCSF seemed like a bad idea so we went to the local ED. They did xrays which didn't show anything knew, and they were able to get on top of my pain reasonably quickly with IV hydromorphone (well, reasonably quickly once they unreasonably slowly established access). Although I shouldn't have been surprised, they suggested I be admitted for pain control. At that point, no sleep, tons of narcs, I was in no position to think clearly but fortunately had other people giving me good advice. They called UCSF and were able to arrange for a transfer that afternoon - which in the scheme of things went

229

waaaaaaayyyyy more quickly and smoothly than I would have anticipated. There was a bit of fucking around once I got to UCSF and I didn't get any more imaging until the following afternoon which meant that instead of going home Tuesday evening I didn't get to leave until Wednesday evening. But in the meantime, I stated radiation for the skull lesion, I met with palliative care who put together a good pain regimen, I had a CT that showed this non-displaced fracture in the left acetabulum, ortho started to get involved (enough to tell me not to put any weight on my left leg for 2 weeks and see them in clinic as the hope is this will heal with conservative management because I don't think there is anything even close to a reasonable surgical solution that anybody in his or her right mind would consider offering or accepting), and I had an MRI (the results of which I don't really know at this point but prelim I was told there wasn't new info as compared to the CT scan). So here's what's up:

1. Skull met - currently being radiated, total of 5 days of radiation, today was day 3 so my last radiation is on Monday. The radiation itself is fairly uneventful but the fatigue will accumulate over time. It will be a few weeks before we know if the proptosis/swelling are going to improve/resolve or if I have to get used to the fact that my face may now just always be fucked up. Fortunately it's not as if is visible to the outside world so that's not a big deal at all. I'm still on high dose steroids and will start a long slow taper at some point after radiation ends.

2. Acetabulum fracture - crutches/walker/wheelchair - no weight-bearing for 2 weeks, follow-up with ortho, hope this can heal conservatively. In the meantime, on around-the-clock oxycodone for pain control - which is working well -

but it is fucking depressing that I can't move around or drive or do much of anything for myself. I am also on denosumab, a monoclonal antibody that inhibits the development and activation of osteoclasts (the cells that eat away bone) and is used to treat osteoporosis and to prevent fractures in people with cancer. It's a monthly infusion I started last month and I will continue with that.

3. Cardiophrenic mass - still a potential problem if/when it gets larger but I have not had a recurrence of the severe pain that brought me to the ED xmas eve.

4. Cancer in general - obviously this shit is going apeshit - at some point over the summer it decided to stop laying low and shit is growing, and growing pretty fast. The only thing to do about this is systemic therapy. I will start the new chemo (trabectedin) next Thursday. This is the 24hour infusion that I get to do at home and should be less unpleasant than the other chemo I've done. I am "looking forward" to starting something systemic in the hopes that it will get this cancer to chill the fuck out. At this point I'm not asking for/expecting/hoping for a magic cure (I know, I know, and up until this point it has been clear from my writing that I've been expecting a magical cure), but if it could just slow this shit down a bit that would be nice. With all these recent, shitty developments I cannot help but feel that I am circling the drain. But I keep trying to remind myself that there is this new, potentially helpful, not insanely unpleasant, treatment I'm about to start that might do something useful. In the meantime, rules about "dogs on the bed" have become a bit more lax and the next time I go out to eat I plan to order one of everything on the menu.

January 14, 2016

Infusing!

Finished my xrt on Monday, tapering off the steroids, got the chemo hookup today. I'm now at home with a little bag of chemo! I go back tomorrow to have them unhook me.

I should point out that now that I'm not putting (much, total nwb is nearly impossible) weight on my left leg I'm not having much pain and am not taking any pain meds. I will also mention that the narcotics fuck with my stomach/bowels so much that I honestly think I am not going to want to take them when I need them again. So much for my plan of becoming an awesome drug addict. Right now eating and drinking delicious things is way at the top of my to-do list and so taking meds that negatively impact that desire and/or ability is way at the bottom of my to-do list. I guess we will see what happens. In the meantime, I plan to eat my face off.

January 15, 2016

Certainly not as rough as it could have been...

Though there is still time. New chemo experience marred by overnight recurrence of flank pain which kept me from sleeping despite another robust round of narcotics. So today I was nauseated and managed to vomit in the car going to get unhooked and coming back from getting unhooked! Thanks to the narcotic haze and those handy little emesis bags it was far less traumatic than it could have been. I got some fluids and ondansetron (considering honoring it with name brand recognition because I ♥☐ it so much) before they unhooked me and those things are always good. And the pain has been much more mild and I haven't needed any pain medicine since this morning. But with not sleeping (from steroid taper from xrt, steroid burst for nausea with chemo, pain) plus narcotics plus chemo it's hard to know what's doing what. Overall, I still feel waaaaaayyyyyy better than I did on day 2 of any other chemo regimens so I am grateful for that.

January 17, 2016

Still feeling reasonably ok

And my appetite is decent. Since "activity is quality of life" (a phrase I got from our vet!) is no longer a phrase that works well for me, I'm converting to "eating is quality of life." Once I can't move around and I can't eat then we have a serious, serious problem.

I neglected to mention that last week we met with my oncologist and I asked him about the not getting radiation post-surgery and the other little ball-dropping issue of a mass detected on a PET scan (not a good way to detect anything in the head) that was written-off as "post-op changes" (even by the neurosurgeon) until 10 days later when I noticed the proptosis and then was sent for an urgent MRI that confirmed the mass. I've raised these issues with my oncologist, radiation oncologist, and the neurosurgeon. The first issue, of not doing xrt postop, is just a clinical decision. The second one is a bit more than an oversight. At this point, I'm not taking a position as to whether either one of them impacts my course or prognosis. But what's more upsetting is the feeling of not having been looked after. And I can't help but feel that it's somewhat ironic that I am negatively impacted by something that, for all the many many ways in which I'm a really shitty and inadequate physician, I am quite confident I would never do - not get the expert (neurosurgeon) to comment on a disturbing finding (mass) on a study I ordered. It does sound like there will be an M+M, which I half-jokingly asked if I could attend. I would love to present myself! I could use all the favorite phrases I hate to describe myself like "pleasant" (which always means "white" or "not white yet unexpectedly pleasant"). But really I'd rather they just have an honest discussion and then I'd like to hear the outcome. My oncologist did point out that my tumor is not behaving the way chondrosarcomas do and it has taken everyone by surprise. Things should be growing over the

234

course of months - but they are growing over the course of weeks.

I will say that I actually do have some hope that this new chemo will do something. I have had decent responses to the chemo in the past and that's when things were growing more slowly. So maybe I'll be the only one who is surprised if this isn't effective. J stopped reading the blog long ago though I don't think anything I put in here would be a surprise to him. I wonder if he knows that I know that this is all way worse for him than it is for me. I have to go through this, physically, but then it's over for me and I don't have to figure out anything after that.

January 20, 2016

Not the shittiest news ever!

We saw the ortho onc guy (OOG) today and he doesn't think that I have much of a fracture - he thinks I may have a whiff of xrt-related osteonecrosis of the femoral head but he's not sure that's the case either. He thinks the films are not super convincing either way, and my pain has improved a lot as I've stayed off the leg. So, I get to weight-bear as tolerated! He suggested going slow, using a cane, but he doesn't think I'm about to break something if I start walking on my leg. This is not the news we were expecting! We didn't even really know what to do with ourselves when he told us! I was just hoping that he wasn't going to tell me to stay off the leg for another 3 months or something.

I did ask if I'm supposed to limit my activity when I have pain - more because it suggests some bad pathology that's going to get worse - or if I can just do what I want as long as I can handle the pain. He acknowledged that activity and quality of life are related and suggested that I spend my time doing things I want like walking the dogs and devote less leg stress to things like washing dishes.

Ha!

J was there when he said that! It really is like I got a note from the doctor that I'm not supposed to do any more dishes!

So, we will see how this goes and then I follow-up with him in 2 months. In the meantime, we will just keep hoping the trabectedin does something useful.

Man, it has been such a long time since a visit to the doctor didn't result in worse news I am not sure how to handle this!

January 20, 2016

So maybe I did a few dishes!

Just because I could!

So there!

January 23, 2016

My hair is falling out!

It's not really supposed to with this chemo - thin but not fall out - I did consider that a big plus - it has been very nice to have hair! But it's only falling out on one side, the side where I had the xrt, so maybe it is from that? But it is not localized to the area where I had the xrt so I don't know wtf is going on.

January 25, 2016

Slight change in plans

Saw my oncologist today - he is pleased with how I've been tolerating the chemo (as am I!). He wants me to do 3 cycles, rather than 2, before the PET scan so as to give this the best shot of working. That means I will start the 2nd cycle early Feb. and the 3rd cycle late Feb. and have the PET scan early March. I'm fine with this plan as the last thing I want is for it to be somewhat unclear as to whether this chemo is effective. If it's not effective, the options are a)look for a clinical trial b)etop/iphos - the inpatient chemo I did last year - not gonna happen and even he isn't really recommending it c)gemcitabine and docetaxel - which at least is an outpatient regimen d)let nature take its course. Fortunately I don't have to make any decisions now.

January 31, 2016

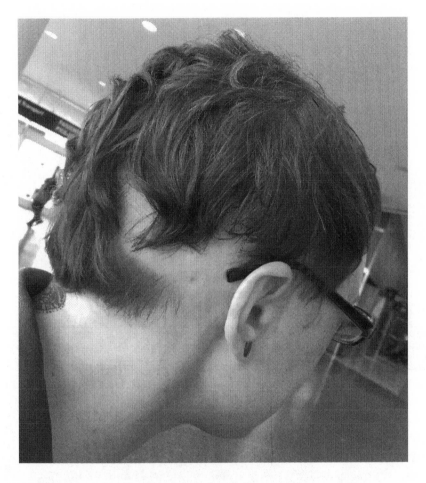

This post-xrt bald spot is no joke! It's gonna be a while before it grows back since apparently hair follicles don't take kindly to being irradiated. In the meantime, I'm considering a tattoo in the space - maybe a rose and the words "fuck you" in a nice script.

Census guy came to the door today. We've been selected to participate in a survey about consumer expenses! All we need to do is record what we spend money on and save our receipts. I feel like we would really throw the numbers off.

"We've noticed a large spike in bakery and chocolatier spending with scones receiving the largest bump from 2015 numbers. Household expenditures on dog treats have also shot through the roof in 2016. We are investigating whether Americans are really spending this large a percentage of their incomes on aged rums."

I told him I really supported the concept but was in the middle of chemo and wouldn't be participating. He, not getting the message, then asked if my husband would record our expenses. I told him that my husband was taking care of me during chemo and would not be participating. He, continuing to not get it, then tried to explain how easy it would be and how little time it would take and he asked if he could leave the materials with us in case we decided to do it. I told him that he was welcome to leave the materials with us if he wanted us to put them in the recycling but we were not going to participate so he might want to hold on to them to bring to another house. He finally realized we weren't going to do it…and then proceeded to take up even more of my time in his attempts to record my not participating. I eventually asked him to make note of my not participating in a way that didn't involve me so that I could get back to living whatever amount of life I have left.

I frequently worry that I'm going to run out of stuff to write about, but then I am reminded that there is no end to the stupid shit that people say and do.

February 4, 2016

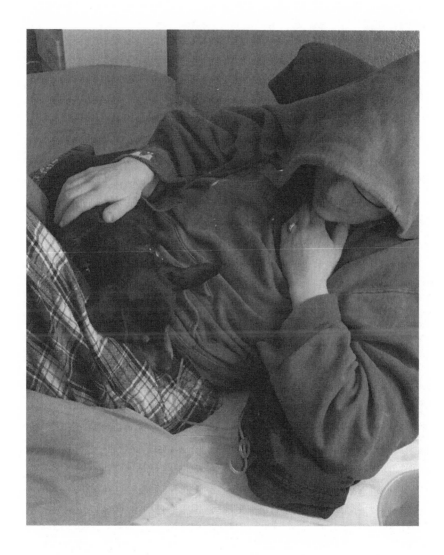

All hooked up, freshly pressed, high-end pajamas on, crime-drama playing, ice cream consumed, small dog and bag o'chemo at my side. She does not normally get in this position. It is pretty clear Cleo knows wtf is going on. Not sure how many times I have to do this before I stop wondering what that noise is (the pump, every few seconds). Feeling ok so far.

February 5, 2016

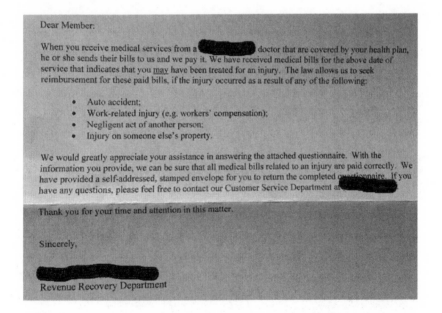

Dear Member:

When you receive medical services from a ▆▆▆▆▆▆▆ doctor that are covered by your health plan, he or she sends their bills to us and we pay it. We have received medical bills for the above date of service that indicates that you may have been treated for an injury. The law allows us to seek reimbursement for these paid bills, if the injury occurred as a result of any of the following:

- Auto accident;
- Work-related injury (e.g. workers' compensation);
- Negligent act of another person;
- Injury on someone else's property.

We would greatly appreciate your assistance in answering the attached questionnaire. With the information you provide, we can be sure that all medical bills related to an injury are paid correctly. We have provided a self-addressed, stamped envelope for you to return the completed questionnaire. If you have any questions, please feel free to contact our Customer Service Department at ▆▆▆▆▆▆▆.

Thank you for your time and attention in this matter.

Sincerely,

▆▆▆▆▆▆▆
Revenue Recovery Department

Hilarious!

This was a visit to a palliative care doctor. Couldn't they check that before they send the letter?

February 24, 2016

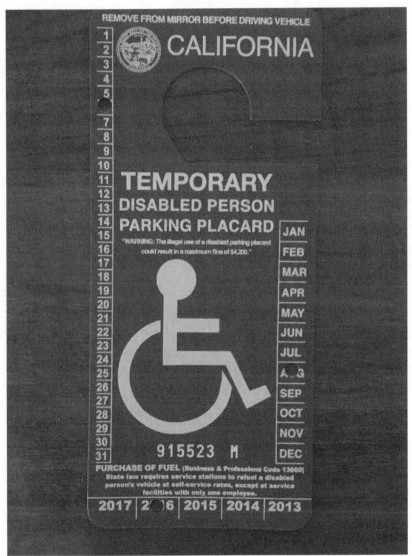

Oh happy day!

February 25, 2016

Best Laid plans...

I'm testing out life mottos - what do you think?

"Curses, foiled again" is also on the short-list.

Supposed to do cycle 3 today but woke up with a sore throat concerned I'm getting a cold so my oncologist said we should delay a week cause chemo+cold = less fun than chemo without cold. The scan will still be mid-March so it doesn't change the exciting "are things still running amok?" determination.

On a totally unrelated note, while skimming the obituaries yesterday (I like to revel in the shittiness of my situation and everyone else at least seems to be able to leave their spouses with a kid or two) and came across the classic "passed away…following a courageous two-year battle with cancer." I sure as fuck hope that nobody says that what I'm doing is either "courageous" or a "battle." A more apt description would be "Rachel tolerated the cancer and the treatment for a while, and then she didn't."

March 2, 2016

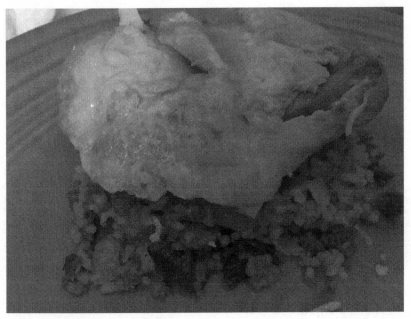

A different kind of chemo…

One that still leaves me with an appetite for things like this -
J's Spanish chicken - brined and stuffed with
couscous/chorizo/spinach/bell peppers/olives/pistachios -
from a recipe he literally dreamed-up. Delicious.

March 5, 2016

Sick and tired

of feeling sick and tired.

This chemo is nothing like the others - but it's not exactly "fun." It is hard to wrap my head around the fact that I'm supposed to hope that it's doing something so that I can feel this way every 3 weeks for the rest of my life. I'm a bit conflicted about that.

At least there are still root beer floats in the world.

March 8, 2016

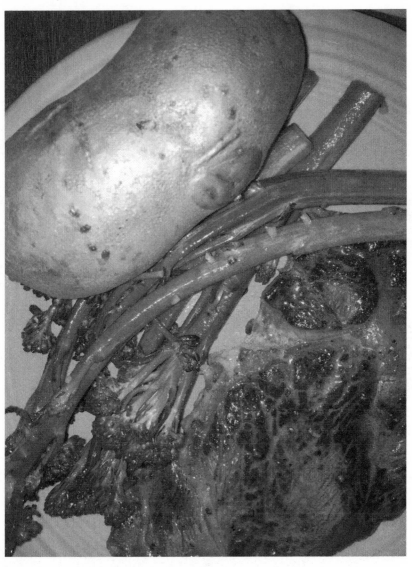

Cancer sucks, chemo sucks, but what doesn't suck is finally having an appetite and craving something specific (steak, potatoes, garlicky broccolini) and having J run to the grocery store to get the ingredients and then whip up a delicious version of what I'm craving. It sure beats the rbf and dorito dinner I had last night.

I hope you all are in agreement that if it's heart disease that gets me that's gonna be hilarious.

March 18, 2016

Not good news!

AKA - bad news!

Scan results are not good - I've got a bunch of new mets (mostly in my skull and chest) which means the chemo isn't working. The older mets are not that dramatically different (in size or metabolic activity) but that doesn't mean much. So we've reached the point where even my oncologist doesn't recommend more chemo. He said that neurosurgery and rad. onc. are discussing whether xrt to the skull lesions would be useful - I should hear back about that within a week or so. But other than that possibility, it looks like I'm done with treatment.

Bright side - I sure as fuck am not spending any more time thinking about my internal medicine boards. I am also done with flossing my teeth (except when necessary - routine flossing is out). And I feel that I'm doing my part in terms of reducing my carbon footprint so I'm not going to spend a lot of time thinking about other ways I can help with that. I'm also trying to convince J that a puppy would solve most of our problems - if our major problem was the absence of a urine smell to our house I think I would have a strong argument.

Dark side - J has taken to playing this song (https://www.youtube.com/watch?v=EzoazPPC7b8). And I guess I'm done with being a doctor. Well, I had a good 13 year run.

Maybe I should have given up sugar??!?!?!?!

March 25, 2016

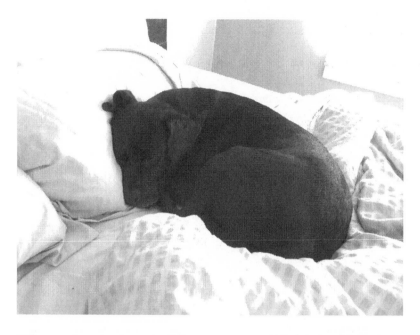

What we've got here is failure to communicate. I said "I'm going to the bathroom, you can get in the bed but don't take my spot." Frankie heard "find the warmest spot in the bed and make yourself at home."

March 29, 2016

I hate vomiting!

But I'm starting to get so good at it I'm wondering if I'm missing my calling if I
Don't keep Working on it. We met with the radiation oncologist yesterday and I vomited while waiting for the appointment, after we met with him and before they did the prelim scans, and then once the appt was over and I was waiting to go home. I carry my own little emesis bags - which are the greatest invention of all time! I want to establish emesis bag containers all over the world (like how they have defribrillators) in airports - it would be at least as handy! It's good to still have goals. Emesis with bags but without borders!

April 8, 2016

I'm not saying Kathy Bates didnt derserve the oscar!

But yesterday I was in bed without any chocolate nearby and my phone wasn't with me - so it was a bit rough!

April 20, 2016

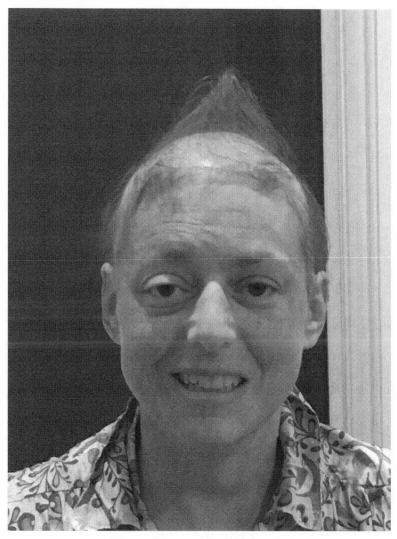

When u r already "wearing a chemise to dinner "there is nowhere to go but up with a stila lip glaze, perhaps in a nice "neutral."

May 2, 2016

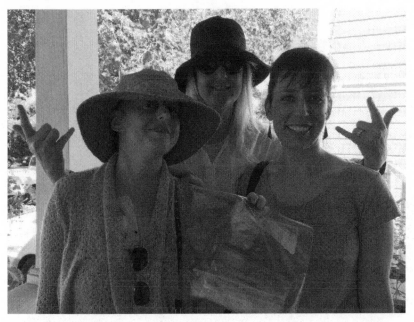

A little Saturday suburb shopping always goes best with a methadone and lorazepam "go kit." And they love it when you fill the syringes on the indoor cream-colored chairs.

May 30, 2016

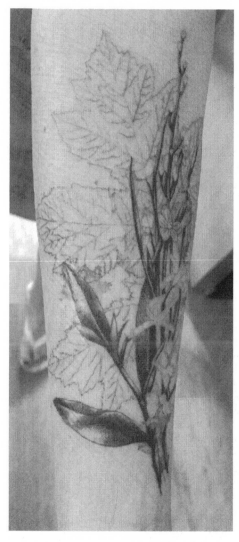

Soooooo overdue for a post - apologies! The whole "chemo not working, more brain mets, seizures, whole-brain xrt, home hospice, etc." has really cramped my style! Though the folks who saw me 2 months ago when I was mostly lying in bed vomiting are pretty impressed with how I am now - I might go out for 2-3 hours, usually for something related to food, and then rest. I don't drive, I don't go out alone, things are pretty different.

The good news is that I happen to be the only person who has ever looked better thanks to the miracles of high-dose steroids. This is all really helping with my hospice as money-maker plan. There has got to be a big market for some hospice-based pornography and I plan to exploit it!

Also, as the astute observers among you may have already astutely observed, I'm getting a new (second) tattoo. This was going to be a ¾ sleeve of my fave California botanicals from our yard in recognition of how much our yard has contributed to my well-being during the whole cancer thing. But that would take about 12 3-4hr sessions over a year and that seems like a goofy thing to do now. So instead I am getting a much smaller subset of plants on my right forearm in about 2 sittings. So I will get it finished in about a month once this first part heals.

June 3, 2016

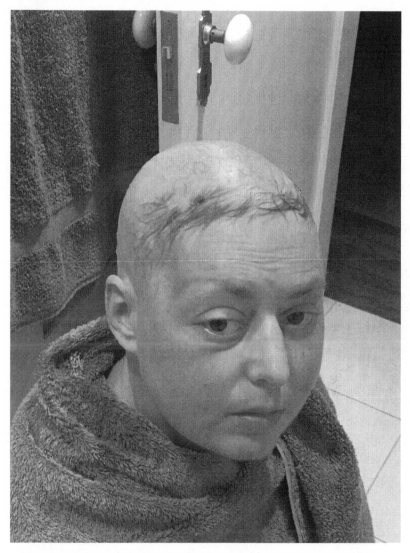

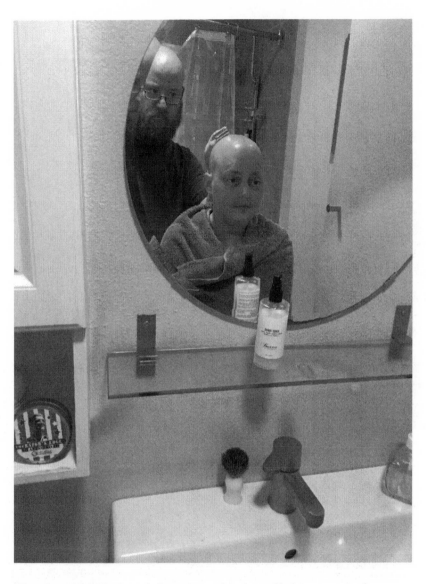

Shaving day! So much better not having all those straggly little hairs around!

June 3, 2016

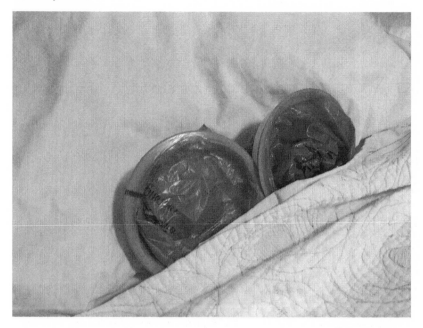

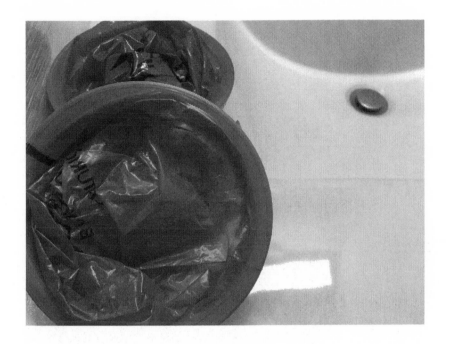

These little emesis bag buddies like to hang in pairs and deserve high thread count sheets and other luxury surroundings. Greatest invention since ondansetron (which we call "dancer" around here).

June 3, 2016

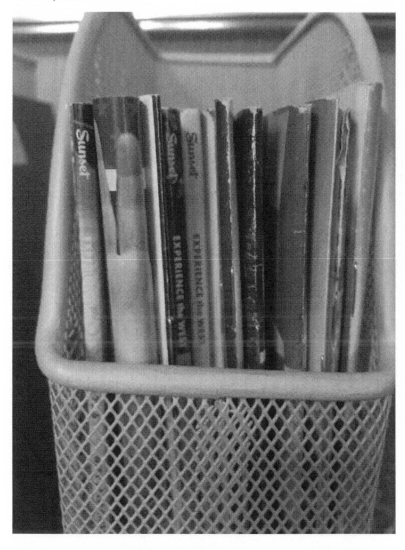

Hospice is busy! I am months behind on The Economist!

June 3, 2016

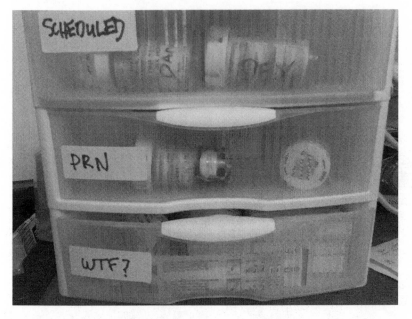

Every MAR should have a WTF section - so handy, so real, so now!

June 3, 2016

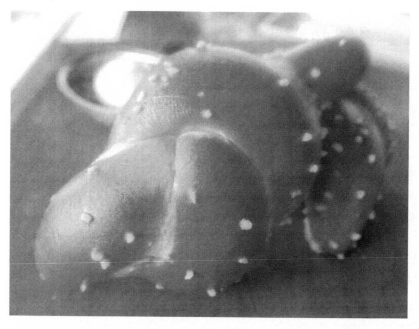

Fresh, artisanal soft pretzels so tasty on an iffy stomach!

June 3, 2016

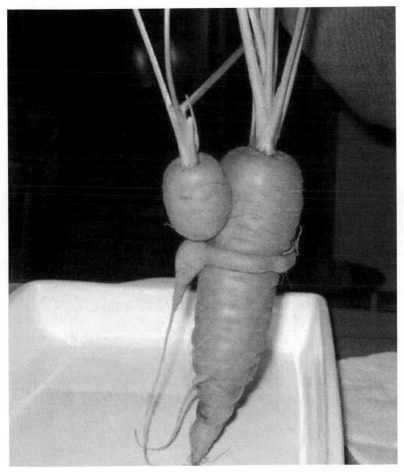

Not our photo but an excellent visual representation of how we are actually getting through this (just pretend there are also a lot of surrounding friends and family carrots - or other supportive fruits and vegetables).

August 16, 2016

The following post has not been evaluated/approved/recommended by any dentists, orthodontists, oral surgeons, or other ENT specialists:

But once you transfer to home hospice, acceptable evening dental care = a root beer float followed by minty ice cream (mint oreo cookie; mint chocolate chip; etc., as long as it's not that fake green stuff!)

August 31, 2016

Until she didn't

Rachel lived with cancer until she didn't. She died the night of August 30. Her parents, her best friend, and I (J), along with our two dogs Cleo and Frankie, sat with her listening to the Giants on the radio.
She went peacefully and painlessly. I held her hand, which was the greatest honor of my life.
Thank you for reading this blog. It meant a lot to her.

August 31, 2016

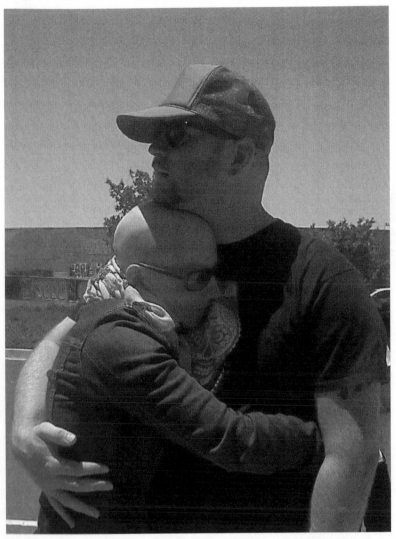

Made in the USA
Lexington, KY
14 March 2018